Health Research Practices in a Digital Context

Health Information Set

coordinated by
Céline Paganelli and Viviane Clavier

Volume 4

Health Research Practices in a Digital Context

Edited by

Laurent Morillon

iSTE

WILEY

First published 2020 in Great Britain and the United States by ISTE Ltd and John Wiley & Sons, Inc.

ISTE Ltd
27-37 St George's Road
London SW19 4EU
UK

www.iste.co.uk

John Wiley & Sons, Inc.
111 River Street
Hoboken, NJ 07030
USA

www.wiley.com

Library of Congress Control Number: 2020938265

British Library Cataloguing-in-Publication Data
A CIP record for this book is available from the British Library
ISBN 978-1-78630-438-4

MIX
Paper from responsible sources
FSC® C013604

Contents

Foreword

This book is the fourth in a set of books entitled "Health Information", coordinated by Céline Paganelli and Viviane Clavier. It is part of the "Health Engineering and Society" collection proposed by Bruno Salgues. Each book is the subject of a specific editorial project designed in close collaboration with its editor(s).

This book focuses on health research practices in the digital environment. It proposes 10 contributions that address, on the one hand, some of the developments in digitally related information and communication practices in the field of health and, on the other hand, some ethical and methodological questions on research carried out in this context. This book is first of all the result of seminars initiated within the health axis of the laboratory of studies and applied research in social sciences (LERASS – EA 827) of Paul Sabatier Toulouse 3 and Paul Valéry Montpellier 3 universities (France). Individual solicitations completed the texts then collected. These proposals were subject to a double-blind evaluation, followed by a constructive process of re-reading and more or less substantial improvements. In this regard, Laurent Morillon, University Professor in Information and Communication Sciences at the University of the French West Indies, LC2S (UMR 8053), warmly thanks the members of the reading committee composed of:

Luc Bonneville, Full Professor, Department of Communication, GRICO, University of Ottawa;

Viviane Clavier, HDR Lecturer in Information and Communication Sciences, GRESEC, Université Grenoble Alpes;

Viviane Couzinet, Professor Emeritus in Information and Communication Sciences, LERASS, University of Toulouse 3;

Jean-Claude Domenget, HDR Lecturer in Information and Communication Sciences, ELLIADD, University of Burgundy – Franche-Comté;

Elizabeth Gardère, Professor of Information and Communication Sciences, MICA, University of Bordeaux;

Sylvie Grosjean, Full Professor, Department of Communication, GRICO, University of Ottawa;

Valérie Lépine, Professor of Information and Communication Sciences, LERASS-Céric, University of Montpellier 3;

Anne Mayère, Professor of Information and Communication Sciences, CERTOP, University of Toulouse 3;

Céline Paganelli, Professor of Information and Communication Sciences, LERASS-Céric, University of Montpellier 3.

Introduction

Health, affirmed as one of the fundamental rights of every human being by the World Health Organization, is at the center of major political, societal, economic, financial, legal, organizational and technological issues. Its developments are indeed occupying a significant place in public debate and media discourse. The French health ecosystem – characterized, among others, by its public status and social security system – is influenced by different environments and actors that modify representations and guide the conduct of activities and practices. For example, the public authorities impose different processes of management, rationalization, standardization or regulation of the healthcare system in order to control (intend to reduce) costs. At the same time, more than ever before, "users" demand customized, reliable and rapid care, and transparency of information. The trend towards "empowerment" invites them to become actors in their own health, both in the prevention and treatment of illness. What is then projected is an idealized figure of a patient – whose experience is now recognized as an expertise – who optimizes his or her disease "trajectory" [STR 92] and care "path" by becoming an "agile" and responsible partner, capable of evaluating the quality of care.

The current "generalized digitization" of society is also influencing the health environment and healthcare actors. The technological environment indeed witnessed the emergence in the 1990s, and then the generalization in the 2000s, of "digital technologies" and in particular the New Information and Communication Technologies (NICTs that have become ICTs). Technical developments have been important in terms of computers, mobile

Introduction written by Laurent MORILLON.

terminals (tablets, smartphones, laptops, etc.), networks (5G, Wi-Fi max, hotspot, fiber, etc.), the Internet of Things, applications, etc. Today, digital technology is omnipresent in everyone's daily life as well as in most professional activities. Thus, "e-health", the use of ICTs for health activities, has brought about profound changes. For example, within dedicated organizations – also responding to the "all-computerized" injunctions of public authorities and certain lobbies – digital technology influences activity and relationships by modulating space and time constraints. It promotes networking, the flexibility of working relationships, the constitution of communities of practice, and the production and dissemination of knowledge. Digital technology is also changing the informational practices (tracing, storing and disseminating) and, more generally, the professional practices of health actors (caring, deciding, coordinating, interacting, etc.). Massive amounts of data produced, distributed and shared by a diversity of (inter)connected devices (applications, software, electronic health records, etc.) contribute to changes in professions, roles and statuses (caregivers, laypeople, academics, experts, etc.), relational spaces (online communities, etc.) and modes of interaction between caregivers and patients. The health Internet has changed relationships with doctors, from scheduling an appointment (online) to a consultation. With information more than ever dematerialized and distributed over the network of networks, even the most specialized information is freely accessible. Many people now consult their doctor with a certain amount of information and advice, without necessarily telling him or her. Whether in terms of research and information sharing or exchanges and controversies, uses are constantly evolving.

However, novelty, especially when it is technical, is often assimilated to modernity and the associated myths are very strong. Digital tools, whether terminals, networks or applications, are thus frequently considered as "magic wands" [PER 89] to better share, communicate or work together. Technology is synonymous with optimization, harmonization, interdisciplinary, speed of execution, collaborative work and organizational rationality. The speeches of its promoters, often caricatured and/or prophetic, invoke the supremacy of digital technology and/or the revolution it would allow. They fuel both the hopes and fears of economic and political actors who do not hesitate to impose the adoption of technologies to "reform".

In this context, research in the humanities and social sciences (HSS) is looking back at the growing importance of digital technology. They understand both the objects and the issues at stake, the logic of use and associated practices, as well as the roles and influences of the devices at work. Beyond the myths, they deconstruct, nuance and sometimes challenge certain preconceived ideas and/or dominant discourses, whether they are technical, managerial or governmental. Since the 1990s, various researchers (Alter, Crozier, Friedberg, Bernoux, etc.) have shown the real uses (from misappropriation to rejection) of technical objects, however efficient they may be. Others (Boutary, d'Iribarne, Gadille, Monnoyer, etc.) have highlighted the costs and drawbacks of ICTs in terms of information security, potential blockages or loss of time. Among the HSS, reflection on ICTs has been rich for the past 20 years and is now well structured in information and communication sciences (ICS). In the field of health, many studies deal, for example, with the influence of digital devices on information retrieval, the appropriation of digital patient records by healthcare teams, the reception of national prevention campaigns, the debates on social networks, etc. Info-communication approaches then go beyond "simple" technical questions.

This book provides an original look at these research works by proposing to focus on research practices. It is a question of taking an interest in "science in the making" which, according to Bruno Latour, is living, uncertain, informal, changing and at the origin of "already made" science that appears in counterpoint as austere, formalist and regulated [LAT 89]. However, it is ambitious to carry out a reflexive return on the modalities of production because if researchers act "in a rather closed field" [GRY 04, p. 151] and their production is accessible, the "factory of science" is not always visible [MON 05]. The object is therefore neither "monumental" science, to use Mondada's expression [MON 05], nor the processes of knowledge creation in the manner of Latour [LAT 89]. The analysis here focuses on a part of the ordinary work of researchers, sometimes not considered because it is regarded as not very noble and/or unproductive. However, more than ever before, beyond ethical behavior and a reflexive quest for rigor, the development of knowledge leads to a detailed explanation of the systems implemented and a justification of the legitimacy of the knowledge developed (LEM 01).

We therefore first invited researchers from the Laboratory for Studies and Applied Research in Social Sciences (LERASS – EA 827), and then those from other French and foreign laboratories, to question their scientific practices through the prism of epistemology, ethics or methodology, once they have grasped digital health. They then conducted an intellectual introspection to shed light on the goals, values and issues of their work, analyzing their posture and approach. By opening their "conceptual toolbox" [MUC 98], they provide a reflexive, even critical, feedback on their methods and techniques, as well as on the choices that have guided the analyses, by revealing elements to be linked. But inviting the scientist to reflect on his or her own practices can induce a form of "implexity". For going back over his/her work and the epistemic path he/she has also taken means accepting the potential for revealing compromises, "tinkering" [LÉV 62], "poaching" [DEC 80] or inconsistencies with the initial objectives.

Contributions to this work come from authors of four nationalities (French, Belgian, Canadian and Mexican) and three disciplines (ICS, of course, as well as sociology and psychology). It brings together 10 contributions and is structured into three parts. The first part, with four chapters, presents, by way of contextualization, some of the changing contexts and info-communication practices related to digital health. These are observations, interviews and sometimes quantitative questionnaires that allow a distanced reading of the phenomena at work.

In the first chapter, Hélène Romeyer looks back over 15 years of work and asks what an ICS researcher can bring to the study of online health, a sector and a professional field characterized by tension and rivalry. In order to avoid a disruptive analysis of digital development in this sector, the author first proposes to deconstruct the idea of a "revolution" generated by digital technology. She favors a study of the chronology of the successive transformations of the health system and notes, among other things, the emergence of genuine content industries specializing in the field of health, a movement towards the privatization of public medical information and attempts to control the legislator. Faced with the multiplication of medical and health information, its ease of access and its continuous nature, Hélène Romeyer then turns her attention to its uses. While the search for information is becoming more permanent and commonplace, she notes that trust in doctors is being maintained, there is interest in the community spaces offered by certain sites and the emergence of new forms of expression.

This study of informative practices is echoed in that of Adrien Defossez. In his chapter, he is particularly interested in the constraints and difficulties faced by sick people in their mobilization of different sources of information in the context of their pathology. To this end, he has initiated about 60 semi-directive interviews with people suffering from cancer. Beyond the information from the doctor, he notes that the patient's health "information system" is made up of digital as well as, and sometimes especially, social resources. Relatives (spouse, relative or friend), when they are called upon, can then occupy an essential place. Whether "professional", "insider" or "lay person", they provide access to differentiated information or resources. But the socio-professional category of the patient offers different opportunities. And while digital resources may then appear as a means of compensating for a "failure" of social resources, their reliability and the ability to use them efficiently may be lacking.

In the third chapter, it is through an autobiographical return that Philippe Marrast takes us to the heart of certain contemporary changes in hospital activity. His interest focuses on hospital rationalization processes and, more particularly, on the implementation of IT tools, such as the electronic health record, to support medical activity. Beyond what can be prescribed, it seeks to know the real and contingent activity of caregivers. This reflection on social practices is taking place in a French hospital specialized in oncology. An original stance in between ICS and computer sciences is developed to question the "sociomaterialities" of work environments. For three years, individual interviews and participant observations enabled him to understand the recomposition of nursing practices and to characterize the transformation of writing modalities. In particular, he notes heterogeneous socio-technical assemblages that require a "fabrication" and a "translation" of information on the part of caregivers and patients. Despite the computerization of patient records, paper remains omnipresent and annotation practices are finally proving to be a part of the complex activity and organization, which is the hospital.

Finally, the first part of this book concludes with a chapter by Silvia Rosa Sigalès Ruiz, Erik De Soir, Claudia Veronica Marquez Gonzalez and Michèle Caria. These researchers propose to analyze online instruction manuals, available in Latin America, to enable volunteers in relief teams to take charge of the psychology of disaster victims (earthquake, flood, terrorist act, etc.). For their qualitative content analysis, they used four criteria: documentary information, pedagogical engineering, mental health intervention protocols and disaster management protocols. For example, they note that the metadata expected for an online educational document is not present; these manuals do not apply the principles of educational engineering; and they have a varying or even partial understanding of intervention protocols in mental health and disaster management. However, while these manuals are freely available on the Internet for any lay person (or general psychologist) wishing to help victims in disaster situations, the implementation of incomplete instructions can become a risk factor for victims and an additional cause of long-term psychological discomfort. To avoid undermining the status of expertise and the legitimacy of their discipline, the authors therefore urge that the scientific validity of the knowledge disseminated on the Internet should be ensured to deal with sensitive situations such as mental health.

In the next two parts of this book, researchers offer reflective, sometimes critical, feedback on their work. In the field of health, moral, ethical and deontological issues are pervasive, numerous and complex. The second part does not list them exhaustively but opens, more modestly, a space for reflection dedicated to this theoretical deontology: moral responsibility of an involved researcher, instrumentalization of science, values and commitments of the scientist, etc. Research activity, as a social practice in fact, introduces researchers into a relationship, sometimes contractual, through which they are confronted with choices that engage its responsibility. Ethics then consists of a set of duties towards each other: research subjects, peers, sponsors, etc. [GOM 96]. In the course of their work, and even more so when they are involved, HSS scientists are committed by their status as researchers, practitioners and citizens [BÉZ 96]. For the health field, if their responsibility seems *a priori* more diffuse than that of medical researchers, for example, the ethical implications are all the more necessary since the object of the research sees the participation of humans who cannot be manipulated as "simple" molecules.

This part opens with the chapter by Aurélie Pourrez, Elodie Crespel, Stéphane Djahanchahi, Olivier Galibert and Benoît Cordelier. Their reflection is based on a research program in Digital Technologies, Information, Communication and Health that mobilizes ethnographic approaches. The project questions the digital mediation of health knowledge and the digitalization of social support between patients and/or caregivers through the observation of online communities. The themes, specificities of the fields, evolving legislative framework, methodological choices and the nature of the comments likely to be collected require, in their opinion, that ethical issues be put into perspective. The questions they ask, which are restricted to empirical and methodological aspects, are varied: Is it necessary to obtain explicit permission from the interviewees to observe and analyze the digital traces of their interactions? Does the researcher-observer have to reveal himself or herself to his or her observers? How can we protect both the observed user-members and the researcher-observers? In order to produce "responsible" knowledge in the field of health in ICS, the authors call for both individual and collective reflective and critical caution, including the subjective as well as intersubjective mobilization of empirical and methodological scientific ethics.

In the following chapter, Emilie Blanc proposes a reflection on both method and ethics. As a social worker in a financial center of La Poste Group, she carried out action research as part of her PhD in ICS. She questions the role of "organizing communication" in the prevention of psychosocial risks related to digital acculturation. In a "therapeutic" aim, research is involved with operational purposes since it aims to transform social practices. Noting the scarcity of presentations and analyses on the actual methodological deployment of action research, the practitioner-researcher proposes to review the method she negotiated with the sponsor and then implemented. In order to act on the prevention of psychosocial risks linked to digital acculturation, she chooses a collective reflection by and for the employees. She uses documentary, quantitative (based on questionnaires) and qualitative (with individual and group interviews) approaches. Finally, the author discusses some of the ethical tensions that arose during the preparation, implementation and reporting of her action research.

In the third and last part of this book, the researchers question the methods they have implemented in projects that addressed health and digital issues. Returning to the method is all the more crucial since scientific fact is not an essence but the result of a process [LAT 99], and it is not so much the object that makes science as the perspective chosen. When in doubt and open to questioning, scientists adopt *a priori* an ad hoc intellectual approach [QUI 88]: they choose from a conceptual toolbox the most relevant techniques, at a given time, according to a specific project. For Moscovici and Buschini [MOS 03], a method is therefore the choice of a way of doing, working and even living. But the relationship to the field and the particularities of the object can induce biases in positions and provisions [BER 06] as well as the emergence of non-rational criteria depending on the actors and their expectations.

In their chapter, Elizabeth Bougeois and Hélène Germain question the interests and limits of interdisciplinary research in the living lab to meet the needs of senior citizens. In a context favorable to "aging well", technologies to palliate loss of autonomy are considered likely to enhance the independence and well-being of older people. However, these devices, which are often designed with a medicalized view of old age, do not always meet the needs of their potential users and can induce fears. It is within the framework of a Living Lab in Health and Autonomy – a device that enables the design of technical solutions for personal assistance with users considered experts – that two collaborative action research projects have been developed. The first aims to collect and analyze the uses and needs of senior citizens in new technologies; the second reconsiders the first study through the prism of the methodological device and what underlies it. Thus, the observation and collection of the responses of the people surveyed redirected the work of the researchers towards a close and set definition of precise needs, based on unique experiences. Similarly, as a result of some difficulties of cross-comprehension in interdisciplinary research work, agreements were reached between researchers in science and technology and researchers in the human and social sciences. But despite these difficulties, interdisciplinarity seems indispensable to the authors in order to design technologies that will support senior citizens in the future.

Dorsaf Omrane and Pierre Mignot present a comprehensive approach to information and communication practices for breast cancer prevention. According to them, prevention, which is inherently complex in nature, requires us to reflect, on the one hand, on how to think globally and, on the other hand, on the methodological framework that will enable us to understand this phenomenon and its info-communication issues. After presenting a summary of the context of organized screening in France – in particular its questioning – the chapter discusses the methodological choices of two projects carried out with a public interest group that implements and coordinates this screening for a French department. The ultimate goal is to offer a series of lectures broadcast to physicians via a secure website. The methodological articulation is original in that it first implements a quantitative approach known as "exploratory", which then allows the construction of a qualitative phase. In the end, quantitative and qualitative analyses of digital social network discourses enrich online ethnographic observations and reveal the existence of social support.

In their chapter, Mylène Costes and Audrey Arnoult advocate for a plural methodological approach in order to initiate research on the place and roles of information sources in "vaccine hesitation". The context is that of a drop in vaccination coverage in France, which would be linked to a climate of mistrust towards vaccination both among the general public and a (minority) fringe of health professionals. Vaccination remains a very controversial topic, especially on digital social networks. The authors first propose to review their exploratory study based on the questioning of 52 people in a pediatric practice. The results guided the questions and the methodological apparatus to be implemented. For the second part of their study, they propose a collection of semi-structured interviews (qualitative) and a lexicometric analysis (quantitative). This choice postulates that qualitative and quantitative are complementary in order to grasp the complexity of the phenomenon. In addition, it allows the researcher's subjectivity in the analysis to be objectified in a certain way. The roles of digital social networks and online forums are part of the focus of the maintenance guide that will be administered.

Finally, in the last chapter, Sophie Dalle-Nazebi proposes to address some epistemological and methodological reflections on qualitative research conducted in sign languages in the field of health. First of all, she sets out the context and two major issues: gaining access to the perspectives of deaf people who use sign language and clarifying the communicative and interactional skills at work in these relationships. The author then discusses some methodological aspects when the languages, media and research methods used are different. It discusses the practical conditions for the production, video recording, transcription and analysis of interviews in French sign language, as well as some of the issues related to the publication of interaction analyses in this language. This reflection finally questions the modalities of participation of researchers and their work of scientific publication. It concludes by encouraging a pragmatic approach to communication issues, taking into account the materiality of communication practices.

References

[BER 06] BERNARD F., "Le laboratoire des sciences de l'information et de la communication. Entre prise, emprise et déprise des pratiques en information et communication", *15th SFSIC Conference, Questionner les pratiques d'information et de communication. Agir professionnel et agir social*, Bordeaux, pp. 1–17, May 2006.

[BÉZ 96] BEZILLE H., VICENTE M., "La recherche en train de se faire : entre rigueur et compromis", in FELDMAN J., FILLOUX J.-C., LECUYER B.-P. *et al.* (eds), *Ethique, épistémologie et sciences de l'homme*, L'Harmattan, Paris, pp. 173–194, 1996.

[DEC 80] DE CERTEAU M., *L'invention du quotidien. 1. Arts de faire*, Gallimard, Paris, 1980.

[GOM 96] GOMEZ L.-E., "Culpabilité et implication", in FELDMAN J., FILLOUX J.-C., LECUYER B.-P. *et al.* (eds), *Ethique, épistémologie et sciences de l'homme*, L'Harmattan, Paris, pp. 48–58, 1996.

[GRY 04] GRYSPEERDT A., "Relations publiques et recherche en communication", *Hermès*, no. 38, pp. 148–154, available at: https://www.cairn.info/revue-hermes-la-revue-2004-1-page-148.htm, 2004.

[KAP 06] KAPITZ C., "L'éthique questionnée par les SIC", *15th SFSIC Conference, Questionner les pratiques d'information et de communication, agir professionnel et agir social*, Université de Bordeaux, pp. 345–351, 10–12 May 2006.

[LAT 89] LATOUR B., *La science en action*, Éditions La Découverte, Paris, 1989.

[LAT 99] LATOUR B., *Politiques de la nature. Comment faire entrer les sciences en démocratie*, Éditions La Découverte, Paris, 1999.

[LEM 01] LE MOIGNE J.-L., *Le constructivisme : vol. 1. Les enracinements*, L'Harmattan, Paris, 2001.

[LÉV 62] LÉVI-STRAUSS C., *La Pensée sauvage*, Éditions Plon, Paris, 1962.

[MON 05] MONDADA L., *Chercheurs en interaction, comment émergent les savoirs*, Presses polytechniques universitaires romandes, Lausanne, 2005.

[MOS 03] MOSCOVICI S., BUSCHINI F. (eds), *Les méthodes des sciences humaines*, Presses universitaires de France, Paris, 2003.

[MUC 98] MUCCHIELLI A., GUIVARCH J., *Nouvelles méthodes d'étude des communications*, Armand Colin, Paris, 1998.

[PER 89] PERRIAULT J., *La logique de l'usage, essai sur les machines à communiquer*, Flammarion, Paris, 1989.

[QUI 88] QUIVY R., CAMPENHOUDT L.V., *Manuel de recherche en sciences sociales*, Bordas, Paris, 1988.

[STR 92] STRAUSS A.L., *La trame de la négociation – Sociologie qualitative et interactionnisme*, L'Harmattan, Paris, 1992.

PART 1

Changes in Contexts and Info-communication Practices Related to the Digital Environment in the Health Field

1

Health and Digital Technology: Reflexive Feedback on Some Works

1.1. Introduction

Working for 15 years on the theme of health from an info-communication perspective, I have been led to study its development on the Internet. We have the opportunity here to look back on this work, on our practices and, beyond that, on our position as researchers in the information and communication sciences (ICS). It is therefore a question of reflecting on the processes used to study the development of e-health and on the concepts mobilized to analyze the results. We will start here by observing the massive presence of e-health; a presence marked by exponential development, a plurality of actors, materials and information. What can an ICS researcher bring to the study of the current state of e-health?

This object, online health, opens the study both on a complex professional field, that of health, a sector marked by its "public" characteristic, and on a sector, that of digital technology, which is still under development, with strong economic stakes and promoted by a number of prophetic speeches. The aim here is to question and sometimes deconstruct a number of ideas or processes about digital technology when applied to health.

First, the framework will be broadened: indeed, the characteristics and issues related to health are such that the situation of online health today cannot be explained solely through digitization. The first element to be

---

Chapter written by Hélène ROMEYER.

deconstructed, therefore, is the idea of a revolution brought about by digital technology. Our first part will show that, in reality, the situation is much more the heir of a long history of political interventionism with important consequences on information. Then, the multiple and high stakes of this situation will lead us to raise the necessity for the researcher to master the digital economy, the functioning of the information and communication industries or the technical processes of the platforms. Finally, if health is developing online it is because it has its users/consumers and therefore there is a use to be analyzed. First of all, the study of these new uses shows a confidence and legitimacy maintained by doctors and then the emergence of new forms of expression. These two elements lead the researcher to deconstruct a certain number of fears about the development of e-health, particularly towards doctors, and to question the real motivations and objectives of Internet users.

1.2. Voluntary changes over the last 50 years

Having worked for several years studying the field of health from an ICS perspective, the observation of a plethora of online information and a dominant discourse on the digital world changing the doctor/patient relationship was relatively quick to emerge. It is, above all, the desire to verify and qualify this phenomenon that has led us to analyze online health. However, once this is established, conducting research on health and the Internet has its pitfalls. Indeed, much work has been carried out by researchers who are primarily interested in the digital world but who are insufficiently familiar with the field of health. This is a nuisance because this situation leads to an attempt to explain phenomena specific to the field of health using digital logic. While the latter obviously have an impact on health, this sector is so specific and complex that the reverse is also true. To ignore it is to be partial in its approach. It is therefore necessary to have an in-depth knowledge of this field, its actors and its characteristics to avoid preconceived ideas or overly rapid assertions. Thus, it is this knowledge of the health professional field that can make it possible to affirm that, in part, the situation of e-health can be explained by a split between medical information and health information, itself the result of nearly 30 years of voluntarist public policies seeking to control medical information only, i.e. that of health professionals. The anarchic situation of e-health is largely due to State action and not to any digital "revolution" (from the Internet to open data).

1.2.1. *An old but partial political desire*

The first difficulty was therefore that of not falling into the dominant discourse of the digital revolution and not falling into the disruptive analysis of digital development in this sector. A researcher is always marked by his/her training. Ours was first constructed in history, which gave us an appetite for continuums rather than revolutions. In fact, when applied to health and the digital world, this makes it possible to replace the technical and political logics: the digitization of health thus follows its computerization under the effect of rationalization policies aimed essentially at controlling costs. Looking back over the history of these developments makes it possible to start again from the specificities of health in France, namely its public nature (in the regalian sense of the term) and the scientific qualification of its information. In doing so, the digitization of health is part of a continuum of proactive public policies.

At the same time, the consumer Internet is developing at a time when the professional health sector is being restructured by various public policies [CAR 02, CON 03]. Faced with the failure of financial control led by doctors themselves, computerization and rationalization of the health sector became reform tools in the 1990s. The chronology of the successive transformations of the health system[1] suggests a long-term movement towards the computerization of both medical and managerial data. The movement to reform the public health system corresponds chronologically to the development of digital information and communication technologies, particularly the Internet. The *Programme d'Action Gouvernemental* (French Government Action Program) for the Information Society (PAGSI), adopted in 1998, clearly indicated that the modernization of information systems in the health and social sector is a priority with a view to "preparing France's entry into the information society" [CAR 00, p. 20]. However, it should be recalled that computerization comprises two essential phases: first, the digitization of information, i.e. the advent of the computer, and second,

1 By way of non-exhaustive examples: supervision of the computerization of the medical sector since 1991 by the Programs for the Medicalization of computerization systems; the law of January 4, 1993, known as the Teulade Law, on the coding of acts and diagnosed pathologies; 2004 implementation of the "*carte vitale*", which governs access to and use of the Social Health Network; subsequently, the Electronic Medical Record or the Personal Medical File complete the computerization of medical data with a curative but, above all, managerial objective.

the extension of digitization to the transport of information, i.e. communication. Additionally, while, in the field of health, the French State has taken charge of and controlled the digitization of information, it has not made the same effort in transporting the information and has to some extent left such exercise to private operators for professional information and to content industries for consumer information. "It is precisely the digitization of information transport that makes it possible to realize the potential for socio-economic transformation that computerization contains in its seed" [RAL 06, p. 146].

The implementation of this system for the circulation of information from medical acts is indicative of a new form of industrialization of the health sector: the digitization of medical data, medical acts and their reports, facilitates the establishment of databases and benchmarking on performance criteria. However, these regulations only affect specialized professional information, not information for the general public. Under the action of public health policies (essentially for accounting purposes), digitization and industrialization of this professional field is therefore taking place.

Having only targeted professionals, a first division is thus established between medical and professional information and health information for the general public. The legislator focused on professional information because its sole objective was to control healthcare spending and thus neglected information for the general public. Private actors, having glimpsed the economic potential of the e-health sector, have taken advantage of this "oversight" to develop tools. It should be noted that the latter, not being interested in medical information or patient health data, are not required to comply with the French legislative framework for medical information. Moreover, as they are not doctors, they are not subject to the supervision of the French Council of Order. As a result, the trend towards opening up to private actors, initiated by the health system reform, is increasing with the development of e-health. What was previously a public and scientific prerogative becomes unregulated and uncontrolled information. However, the evolution has not been limited to changes in the organization of work: it is the development of the use of information and communication techniques for and by professionals, and for and by patients, which is taking hold on a permanent basis. It is thus the only profession that has been forced by the legislator to computerize.

Ultimately, an unprecedented “explosion” of medical and health databases and information is occurring. All this data and information is now accessible to everyone, all the time, as long as you have an Internet connection. Indeed, during this rationalization effort, the network of networks has developed and, thanks to several high-profile political-legal cases and widely publicized militant actions, health issues have gained public space: contaminated blood, asbestos, the “mad cow” crisis, the Distilbene affair, H1N1, etc. [ROM 10]. The emergence of health issues, public action for rationalization and media coverage have thus multiplied the discourse and therefore the information relating to health. The production and dissemination bodies have increased to the point where the supply of information is overwhelming[2]. And the latter has very different statuses: provision of information, scientific reports, commercial strategies for such and such medicines, advice, practical information, online consultations, archives, free services, paid services, etc. True content industries have specialized in the health field.

1.2.2. *Coexistence of two types of information: medical and health information*

It is as a result of this development of public policies and the development of the Internet for the general public that the transition from medical, scientific and official information to health information for the general public is taking place [ROM 15]. Healthcare in France has always been conceived as a matter of public domain. Therefore, medical information is public information, in the strong sense of the term. The specificity of the data gives it its second characteristic: it is scientific, i.e. it meets standards of production and validation by a community before dissemination. As public information, it is fully in line with the way in which public policies operate; as scientific information, it must meet the precise evaluation and dissemination criteria of the scientific community before being addressed to the general public. However, it is this health information that will undergo a complex publicization movement: not only are elements that are eminently privately relevant publicized, but, above all, patients, their relatives or associations produce information via

2 In December 2018, 32.6 million Internet users visited at least one health/well-being site (Médiamétrie, 01/30/2019). All this for 53 million Internet users counted each month according to the 2018 Internet year balance sheet (Médiamétrie, 02/14/2019).

information–communication techniques without going through the medical or scientific sphere. Since the mid-1990s, in France, the production of health information has no longer been the prerogative of the medical sector or the public sector (State). And this digital information is now accessible in a volume and at a speed never experienced before, according to an informationalization perspective [MIE 99].

More specifically, two types of information coexist: medical information, traditionally produced by specialists and meeting the criteria and functioning of public scientific information, and a new category of information, intended for the general public, which is disseminated on the Internet. This information, which we have described as health information [ROM 08, ROM 12], is produced by both the medical sector and the State. This cohabitation creates a tension between health professionals attached to specialized professional medical information, which is highly supervised and regulated by the State, and industrialists or content companies wishing to develop health information for the general public, which is not subject to any control. Paradoxically, while several studies are constantly questioning the reliability or validity of this information [NAB 02, BOU 03], Internet users seem to have integrated it, know how to direct their research and are developing a very different use of these two types of information [PAG 10].

Public medical information is therefore marked by a movement towards privatization. This expression includes the intervention of actors from the economic sphere (Astra Zeneca, Airmedis, Medcost), as well as a movement of privatization by individuals themselves, with the use of medical information in the private sphere and for strictly individualized purposes. This privatization movement is finally accompanied by forms of commodification of public information. This is becoming a commercial issue in more ways than one.

The need to study the current situation not as evidence of a rupture or revolution but rather with some historical depth becomes obvious. It is the history of public policies in France that, by focusing on professional information and leaving the field open to publishers of consumer content, partly explains the situation of online health, and not the intrinsic revolutionary power of the Internet.

1.3. Significant issues

The second difficulty facing the ICS researcher is the complexity of the issues revealed by the massive presence of health on the Internet: economic issues of course for entrepreneurs seeking profitability; professional issues also for doctors who have informed patients coming to them, and who, caught between the injunctions of the Council of the Order and the attraction of online collaborations, find it very difficult to situate themselves. Professional issues, also, for science journalists deprived of the monopoly of the status of information producer.

All these issues create tensions and rivalries. In fact, today, we are faced with a situation of a plethoric and anarchic presence of health sites, a market that has become very competitive and, finally, the first attempts at control on the part of those who feel overwhelmed.

1.3.1. *Economic and professional issues*

The stakes of the technological, economic, political and societal changes at work are of different orders, all interdependent. First of all, there is increased commodification, while the broadening of the information offer leads to differentiated consumption, thus accentuating individualization which in turn reinforces diversification [MIE 00, BOU 08]. The economic stakes are therefore high. Then, a process of self-mediation [MIE 00] develops, since information–communication techniques and networks favor inter-individual relations, without intermediaries. Finally, companies specializing in content production have entered the health sector. This is the case of Linternaute.com/sante (www.l'internaaute.com/sante), which went online in 2006 and is owned by the Benchmark group, which specializes in publishing content for the Internet (owner, among others, of Copain d'avant or Le Journal du net). Doctissimo (www.doctissimo.fr), on the other hand, has had a different trajectory: first founded in 2000 and developed by a specialist in publishing medical content (Medcoste), which has become the flagship health website in France, it was acquired in 2008 by the Lagardère Active group, and, in 2018, by the TF1 group. In 2008, *Doctissimo* was the most visited health website in France. After this date, it has become difficult to accurately measure the site's audience because it is provided at the level of the groups in various rankings, Lagardère then TF1, and not systematically broken down by site only.

Major media groups have therefore invested in health information: the advertising manna associated with the Internet and the presence of giant databases of Internet users, potential buyers, are, no doubt, related to this. And the movement is international: for example, Axel Springer, a German press group, owns Sante-az.aufeminin (www.sante-az.aufeminin.com), which has been operating since 2005. As we can see, the economic stakes and merger/acquisition movements offer an additional difficulty to the good understanding of e-health: the need to master the digital economy, and beyond that the political economy of communication, as well as the functioning of the culture, information and communication industries.

From the point of view of the professional stakes, two seem immediately obvious: one for the doctors present on these sites, and the other for the journalists as regards the production of information. The presence of physicians on consumer websites, beyond the effect of scientific legitimization, also responds to strategies by operators and physicians to circumvent legal provisions. These doctors are thus constantly referred to as "collaborators" or "experts" and their activity is qualified as "advice", "opinion" but never as consultation (prohibited by law). The communication possibilities offered by the creation of new digital media do not abolish the legal and ethical obligations and responsibilities of physicians who use them. For example, section 75 of the Code of Medical Ethics states that any medical advice, service or information must be provided only by professionals qualified in the medical specialty in question.

In 1999, the *Conseil national de l'Ordre des médecins* (French National Council of the Order of Physicians) set up a commission on information technology and new technologies, which has published numerous works on this subject. In addition to these documents, in February 2001, the basic clauses "that should be included in any contract between a physician and a company involved in the medical Internet field" were published. The Order of Physicians reminds us that medicine is a personal activity that is practiced from person to person. If online consultation is prohibited, it is because it denies two fundamental principles of the profession: consultation, a unique colloquium between the doctor and the patient, and the fact that medicine is practiced by a person who takes personal responsibility for it. It should be noted that on October 26, 2010, a decree published in the *Journal Officiel* authorizes consultation by Internet for doctors who are licensed in France. This principle has been partly called into question since 2017 with the implementation of remote consultation terminals to compensate for medical deserts.

Physicians are thus offered addressable Internet spaces in the form of websites, such as information sites, email sites, online study sites, or even sites capable of managing several or all of these different functionalities. One example in this category is the Santepratique site (www.santepratique.fr), online from 2008 to 2018 and managed by IDS Santé SA, a company that produces health content for doctors' offices and pharmacies[3]. However, doctors and insurance companies are also present. Thus, Docteurclic (www.docteurclic.com), created in 2001, is owned by Medsite, a limited company run by doctors, and E-santé (www.e-sante.fr), created in 2002, belongs to a group of mutual funds, including *Garantie Mutuelle des Fonctionnaires* (GMF), one of the oldest mutual insurance companies in France (1934).

1.3.2. *A plethora of information*

Diversity of information, plurality of actors, important economic stakes, differentiated legislation: everything comes together to provoke an exponential presence of e-health. It is now becoming difficult to find our way around this nebula. The third difficulty is for the researcher, on the one hand, to try to create a typology of e-health, and, on the other hand, to analyze the attempts to control this information by public authorities and the Council of the Order.

Health sites can be classified according to five main types: first, Internet users can find few sites or spaces that are accessible only to professionals; second, institutional sites (French ministries, French National Institute for Prevention and Health Education, French National Cancer Institute, French High Authority for Health, etc.) can be classified according to the type of site they are visiting. There are many more commercial sites (insurance, medical equipment, food supplement, pharmaceutical industry sites, etc.); there are also many more associative sites, which are well developed; and finally, there are information sites for the general public. Accessibility, target audience and type of information vary according to these different categories. The first category is the only one with restricted access. The information is professional and medical. All the other categories are available for free access. However, the information disseminated oscillates between public information, which is produced and controlled by public

3 Since taken over by web insights, a content publishing company.

services, market information and a diversified supply of information. Association sites and general public health sites fall into the latter category with a combination of public health information, medical information, advice, practical life, support and games/quizzes. This hybridization of content is a difficulty for the researcher, which is undoubtedly what also makes the success of these sites. All of these sites, apart from the first category, target all citizens who use the public health system, health professionals, patients or their families. For the two categories engaged in content hybridization, the target audience is threefold: members of associations, often patients and their families, as well as health professionals and the media. Table 1.1 illustrates this typology and provides a framework for the researcher's analysis.

	Access	**Type of information**
Professional sites	Restricted	Professional information Medical information
Institutional sites	Free	Public health information Prevention
Merchant sites	Free	Market information Marketing Advertising
Associative sites	Free	Public health information Medical information relayed Medical information produced Advice, practical life
Health information sites for the general public	Free	Medical and health information Public health information Market information Counseling Forums – life stories Quizzes/games

Table 1.1. *Typology of e-health in France*[4]

4 The first version of the typology was published in [ROM 12]. It is updated and clarified here. This article was based on a study of eight consumer health websites.

The distinction introduced in France in the 1990s between medical information and health information, described in the first part of this paper, is perfectly reflected in this table. The consumer health sites, the least controlled by public authorities and the most subject to a competitive market, then embody a hybridization of the other four types of existing sites.

The plurality of this information and that of its producers leads to a diversity of interests defended by each and every one of them. Health information for the general public is not intended to be of general interest and does not aim to disseminate prevention information, unlike institutional (Inpes, INCa, Inserm, etc.) or associative sites. These types of sites defend commercial interests and are not subject to the same control as sites where public and scientific information can be found. This situation has led the legislator, the High Authority for Health (HAS) and the Council of the Order to propose methods for controlling online health information for the general public.

1.3.3. *Attempts to control*

In 2004, the legislator entrusted the HAS with the mission of "determining the rules of good practice to be respected by sites dedicated to health"[5]. The Health On the Net (HON) Foundation was entrusted with the implementation of the system by HAS experts. The latter created the specifications of the HON standard, which, rather than guaranteeing the content, focuses on framing the container by imposing principles of transparency on publishers. Labeled sites must clearly display their sources of funding, indicate the source of the information disseminated and the quality of the authors, and ensure that advertising is recognizable and cannot be confused with editorial content. Finally, they must ensure and preserve the confidentiality of personal information given on the site. The HON claims 6,000 labeled sites[6]. This is not much compared to the 43,000 resources (including 10,000 sites) deemed to be of quality by the Rouen University Hospital and indexed for 10 years on CISMeF.org (catalogue and

5 Article L 161-38 of law no. 2004-810 of August 13, 2004 (decree of 10/26/2004).

6 https://www.hon.ch/HONcode/Patients/index_f.html.

index of French-language medical sites)[7]. It is also insufficient to measure the intrinsic quality of the information transmitted online.

We may wonder about the real role of this certification: since it is based on a voluntary approach and has no system of sanctions, some sites have no interest in requesting it. It ends up becoming a marketing tool, useful for the least known sites, and then playing the role of legitimization, and useless for sites already enjoying a good reputation. Thus, sites owned by the Lagardère, TF1 and Springer groups do not display the HON standard.

Finally, this HON standard is a communication and posting action rather than a control element of the information disseminated by the general public information sites. If elements are indeed provided to Internet users on certified sites, they are well hidden in the spaces outside the active page, in the headings "Legal notices" or "Ethics", but not directly accessible in full page. None of the eight sites analyzed claims that professional journalists produce this information. All mention working with one or more physicians. However, where data are available on the distribution between journalists and doctors, it is very much in favor of the latter. Thus, for the E-santé site, while 28 journalists are mentioned as working on the production of the articles, more than 100 doctors are listed as collaborators.

Internet users therefore have access to diversified, medically validated and regularly updated content on the general public information sites, but these are not the spaces they visit, according to the results of the survey conducted by the Council of the Order (which cross-checked the results of the survey we conducted in 2006–2007). Clearly, these are the community spaces that Internet users frequently visit, i.e. the sites where they can exchange ideas, play games and take tests. It is therefore the social aspects that seem to interest Internet users more than the information content, which is what health professionals and public authorities are trying to control.

1.4. New uses

Over the last 20 years or so, health has therefore undergone a slow process of computerization and then media coverage. The first consequence was the multiplication of information, the ease of access to it and its

7 http://www.chu-rouen.fr/cismef/projet-cismef/a-propos/.

continuous nature. These characteristics then upset the traditional framework of the singular colloquium. It no longer pits a single professional who holds the information against a supposedly ignorant patient, but proposes a situation in which the two discuss (sometimes debate) on the basis of information that they jointly hold [TAB 19].

1.4.1. *Continued confidence in physicians*

Given the success of online health information and the inability to control it, the Council of the French Medical Association invited experts, institutions and journalists on May 4, 2010 to discuss the evolution of online health information. At this meeting, the results of a study carried out in 2010 by Ipsos were presented[8]. These data largely echoed a survey we conducted in 2006 and 2007[9] on similar themes. In four years, the results remained fully compliant despite the exponential development of digital practices and the sites or other applications available. They are also in line with the various surveys carried out in recent years: all these studies show the continued development of online information searches by the French; however, the latter also constantly reaffirm their confidence in their doctor for the validity of health information. Thus, contrary to many of the speeches produced at the turn of the millennium, Internet users are perfectly aware of the fluctuating reliability of what they find online and in no way substitute the Internet for their doctor. Internet users continue to consider that the best source of health information remains their doctor (83% in 2006–2007, 89% in 2010 and 56% in 2019). What is changing is that the Internet comes second (after doctors) among sources of information for Internet users in 2010, whereas the Internet was not cited as a legitimate source of information in 2006. In 2019[10], while doctors are still popular for 56% of the French, search engines (31%) are now ahead of websites (23%), but pharmacists (43%) have slipped between doctors and the Internet. In addition, the share of Internet users trusting the information available on the Internet increased from 48% in 2006 to 74% in 2010. It is therefore undeniable that the search for health-related information on the Internet is

8 Survey "the consequences of Internet use on patient–doctor relationships", April 2010 (a sample of 1014 people).

9 Questionnaire survey and interviews with users of the Doctissimo forum between 2006 and 2008 (103 questionnaires and 18 interviews).

10 Statista 2019, IPSOS survey.

becoming more widespread and commonplace; similarly, the doctor remains the preferred reliable source, but at the same time mistrust of online content is tending to fade.

Doctors, for their part, seem to find it difficult to accept this new situation of the singular colloquium where the patient is no longer passive and arrives with a certain amount of information. Is it a fear of being dispossessed of power (the sole holder of knowledge)? The one about being questioned? Probably in part, or at least at first. However, what emerges from the various interviews conducted with doctors is[11] rather a weariness to note that the time of consultations is getting longer because of these discussions and that they must now deny, correct, explain or deconstruct the information gleaned by patients on the Internet. Inevitably, in a context of doctor shortages, in a situation where the number of daily consultations is increasing, this creates tensions. Thus, in 2010, as in 2006, Internet users were reluctant to tell their doctor that they had conducted research on the Internet: 63% of them hid it in 2006 and 65% in 2010. While Internet users said they feared the doctor's hostile reaction to the Internet in 2006, 31% of 2010 Internet users said they had experienced negative feelings. It is a complex situation that is taking shape: patients who inform themselves on the Internet having taken the measure of the information available, who keep all their confidence in their doctor, but, patients who do not venture to reveal to him or her that they have been on the Internet, while at the same time nourishing the consultation of the information in their possession.

1.4.2. *Beyond information: life stories and testimonies*

This paradox is partly explained by the study of discussion forums and surveys on the motivations of Internet users: the latter are not primarily interested in information. What they like is the link through the community spaces that Internet users frequent, i.e. the sites where they can exchange, share, move, sympathize and advise. The real change in e-health lies in the emergence of this non-expert, non-professional voice. This movement to publicize an ordinary word is not specific to the media and must be seen in the context of a broader social movement, that of "forms of citizen involvement in decisions that concern them" [ROS 06, p. 301]. In the field

11 A series of 22 interviews were conducted with doctors in charge of information services in various French hospitals between January and August 2006.

of health, the situation is particular because – as we have pointed out above – this information was traditionally public (emanating from the State or major public research bodies) and scientific (requiring a precise knowledge base and validation circuits specific to this sphere). In this setting, patients never had a direct voice. Others have always spoken for them. It is precisely from this niche (individual, direct and testimonial expression) that the content industries are seized. This investment was motivated first and foremost by the media status of health [MAR 10], which guarantees its success in terms of audience ratings. This is then favored by the absence of a binding legislative framework, unlike professional information, which greatly facilitates its development. This investment is finally favored by the trends towards individualization and dematerialization of media, as well as by the massive use and development of information–communication techniques [GROS 07, CAR 02], which are now winning over the general public. Moreover, health, which refers to a large extent to intimacy, is thus perfectly attuned to the practice of anonymity and the use of pseudonyms specific to the community Internet. Generating consubstantial empathy, it provokes interaction almost naturally. This characteristic is particularly clear through the emergence of new forms of words: life stories and testimonies. However, the phenomenon that the Internet underlines with regard to the expression of the sick (and their entourage) is the emergence of testimony (or life story). The content analysis we conducted of the Doctissimo forum reveals that testimonials account for about 50% of the exchanges. The forum is becoming more and more like a real virtual community, which is united by a common trait: illness, a need for information, suffering. It is not a place where you come for information. Moreover, many of the replies remain unanswered.

The digitization of this ordinary expression, of the word of the sick, has shaken the status of testimony. We have measured it through several studies on the emergence of this word in traditional media as well as on the Internet. In Table 1.2, we summarize the results of this research, one dealing with health programs on television, through which the issue of the use of testimonials was analyzed, and the other dealing with non-professional speech on the Internet and focusing on the development of life stories[12]. This table categorizes both the aims, tone and different statuses of the testimony according to the media and the time period.

12 [ROM 07] and [ROM 12].

	Illustrative testimony	Argumentative testimony	Informative testimony
Appears	19th Century (popularization) until today	Mid-1980s to present day	Late 1990s to present day
Supports	Traditional press (health and science sections) Television and radio	Television and radio (talk show, night show) Traditional press (society and politics section)	Internet (forum) Social networks Blogs
Aims at	Outreach Pedagogy	Evidence Debate/charge	Individual expression Solidarity – empathy Informative
Tone	Didactic Technical and specialized	Compassionate Controversial	Emotive Intimate Togetherness Informative
Status	Example	Argument	Constitutes the message

Table 1.2. *Place and role of testimonials in health information*

Armed with the vast amount of information available online, and fed by the multiplication of testimonials, patients are now going to their doctor's office or making decisions about their health (vaccination, for example). The doctor is therefore no longer the only actor in the health of individuals. These new uses of health information, the multiplication of actors, types of information and media should lead us to think of the production of health information as a "chain of cooperation" [BEC 88] between ordinary Internet users, information professionals and health professionals. In fact, in the marketing operation of these sites, the argument of cooperation and the promise of community spirit are at the root of strategies to capture the attention of Internet users. However, the scarcity of this attention is the object of multiple strategies. Beyond this promise of cooperation (collaborative spirit), it is clear today that the production of health-related information involves a complex chain of cooperation comprising scientists, journalists, web actors, patients, associations, activists, health and political personnel.

1.5. Conclusion

Through this reflexive feedback, the info-communication study of online health imposes several saving postures on the researcher.

First of all, it is necessary to study the health situation not in terms of digitization, but rather on the basis of a good knowledge of the field of health, its history, its actors and its functioning, in order to envisage the introduction of digital technology. It is therefore a question of avoiding the discourse of the "revolution" generated by digital technology and not falling too quickly into a disruptive approach. In this respect, operating over a long period of time, thinking about innovations in terms of a continuum rather than a rupture, analyzing actors' strategies, in short, working on the notion of "social logic" as defined by Bernard Miège [MIE 04] is more relevant.

Second, the very important and complex issues at stake, whether economic, technical, professional, scientific or societal, make it necessary to acquire several analytical tools and to enrich one's own disciplinary "toolbox". How can we understand the evolution of e-health without mastering – even partially – the digital economy or the balance of power and strategies of players in the communication industries? How can we understand the emergence of new forms of expression without placing them in broader movements such as the questioning of experts, new social movements, the development of information and communication technologies, etc.? How can we finally work on health in France without taking up the whole range of public policies in this area and without analyzing the politicization of health?

In conclusion, to study health online for an ICS researcher is to accept incompleteness. Changes are at work, interactions are numerous, the stakes are high and the dynamics are still ongoing. None of these interacting elements, taken in isolation, is sufficient to understand the situation. It is the balance of power between them and the ongoing adjustments that informs the e-health situation.

1.6. References

[BEC 88] BECKER H., *Les mondes de l'art*, Flammarion, Paris, 1988.

[BOU 08] BOUQUILLION P., *Les industries de la culture et de la communication. Les stratégies du capitalisme*, PUG, Grenoble, 2008.

[BOU 03] BOURRET C., "la santé en réseaux", *Études*, vol. 399, no. 3, pp. 175–189, 2003.

[CAR 00] CARRE D., PANICO R., "Les enjeux socio-médicaux de la modernisation de la santé", *Terminal*, no. 82, pp. 7–30, 2000.

[CAR 02] CARRE D., *Régulation sociale de la diffusion des TIC*, HDR, Stendhal University, Grenoble 3, 2002.

[CON 03a] CONVERT B., DEMAILLY L., "Le savoir médical et sa mise en scène sur le net", *Terminal*, no. 89, pp. 65–76, 2003.

[CON 03b] CONVERT B., DEMAILLY L., "Internet et les professions de santé: le problème de la consultation à distance", *Réseaux*, no. 120, pp. 241–269, 2003.

[MAR 10] MARCHETTI D., *Quand la santé devient médiatique. Les logiques de production de l'information dans la presse*, PUG, Grenoble, 2010.

[MIE 99] MIEGE B., TREMBLAY G., "Pour une grille de lecture du développement des techniques de l'information et de la communication", *Sciences de la Société*, no. 47, pp. 9–22, 1999.

[MIE 00] MIEGE B., *Les industries du contenu face à l'ordre informationnel*, PUG, Grenoble, 2000.

[MIE 04] MIEGE B., *L'information-communication, objet de connaissance*, de Boeck Supérieur, Brussels, 2004.

[NAB 02] NABARETTE H., "L'internet médical et la consommation d'information par les patients", *Réseaux*, no. 114, pp. 249–286, 2002.

[PAG 10] PAGANELLI C. *et al.*, "Dynamiques interactionnelles et rapports à l'information dans les forums de discussion médical", in MILLERAND F., PROULX S., RUEFF J. (eds), *Web social. Mutation de la communication*, Presses universitaires du Québec, Montreal, 2010.

[RAL 06] RALLET A., "Technologies de l'information et de la communication. Enjeux de société", in DE OLIVESI S. (ed.), *Sciences de l'information et de la communication. Objets, savoirs, disciplines*, PUG, Grenoble, 2006.

[ROM 07] ROMEYER H., "La santé à la télévision: émergence d'une question sociale", *Questions de communication*, no. 11, pp. 51–70, 2007.

[ROM 08] ROMEYER H., "TIC et santé: entre information médicale et information de santé", *Revue Tic&société*, available at: http://revues.mshparisnord.org/lodel/ticsociete/index.php?id=365, 2008.

[ROM 10] ROMEYER H., Les discours médiatiques du cancer, Post-doctorate report for the Institut National du Cancer, 2010.

[ROM 12] ROMEYER H., "La santé en ligne", *Communication*, vol. 30, no.1, available at: http://journals.openedition.org/communication/2915, 2012.

[ROM 15] ROMEYER H., "Publicisation et médiatisation des sujets de santé", *Cahiers de l'ILSL*, no. 42, pp. 153–181, 2015.

[ROS 06] ROSANVALLON P., *Le modèle politique français*, Le Seuil, Paris, 2006.

[TAB 19] TABUTEAU D., "Santé digitale", *Les Tribunes de la santé*, vol. 60, no. 2, pp. 5–6, 2019.

2

Social and Digital Resources: The Hindered Information Practices of Cancer Patients

2.1. Introduction

In an article from the late 1990s, Robert Kraut and his colleagues contrasted sociability on the Internet with more traditional forms of sociability with close friends and family, considering that the development of the former was taking place at the expense of the latter [KRA 98]. While the results of this article have since been widely questioned [CAR 14, TUB 12], it is frequent to see this type of opposition resurfacing between activities based on the use of digital tools and those that would do without them.

From this point of view, the practices of health actors, both patients and professionals, have constantly been questioned. In view of the development of e-health, the information practices of patients, in particular, are the subject of numerous discussions within social science disciplines such as sociology and information and communication sciences. Work on this subject seeks, above all, to measure the uses and preferences of patients in terms of sources of information. Much less attention has been paid to the difficulties that patients encounter in mobilizing these different sources of information and using them to their advantage in the management of their condition. In this

---

Chapter written by Adrien DEFOSSEZ.

chapter, we focus the discussion on these thwarted informational practices by presenting, on the one hand, the constraints that patients face in mobilizing their close circle of family and friends in the context of the disease, and, on the other hand, the difficulties they encounter in obtaining information through the Internet. To do so, we rely on a survey using semi-structured interviews that we conducted between 2010 and 2014 with approximately 60 cancer patients with various socio-demographic characteristics. Six out of 10 of the patients interviewed were women. The patients seen were aged 23–82 years, with a median age of 61 years. With regard to the age of the patients, most of the respondents were retired. If we consider the last job held, half of the individuals belonged to the professions and socio-professional categories of workers and employees and only 10% of the patients corresponded to higher positions. It should be noted that the vast majority were still receiving care at the time of the interview, while 12 people had completed treatments. We found in our population extremely varied types of cancer (lung, prostate, uterus, pancreas, etc.) although breast cancer was mostly represented (about one-third of the patients encountered). Three-quarters of the interviews were carried out in the hospital establishments taking care of the patients (two different establishments), while the others were conducted in people's homes. The stories of disease trajectories collected during these interviews focus on the resources sought by patients throughout their journey.

The interviews were transcribed and are subject to qualitative and quantitative analysis. Indeed, a database was built up from this narrative material in order to carry out statistical processing concerning the resources sought by patients and the means mobilized to obtain them. The chosen analysis method was thus based on a relational chain approach [GRO 11], which specifically studied the way in which people managed, or not, to mobilize and "benefit" from the various contacts and devices available in their environment. This approach made it possible to quantify the resources sought, the means of obtaining them and to carry out a qualitative analysis of access to resources by considering the mobilization of the relational entourage and the mechanisms within a social process, in this case the trajectory of the disease, in order to better understand the experience lived by the individual.

2.2. Patients and information

In terms of information retrieval, a distinction can be made between social resources and digital resources. The distinction made here is not in the content of the resource itself, but in the way in which it is obtained. It can thus be considered that some information sought by patients can be obtained through their relational environment (social resources), while others are accessible through devices, for example digital devices such as the Internet (digital resources).

Studies conducted on the issue of patient information generally highlight the benefits that individuals derive from the information obtained: a review of the literature on the need for information among cancer patients indicates that it enables patients to participate more in decision-making about their disease, reduce their anxiety and better manage their illness [RUT 05]. From the time the cancer is diagnosed until the end of treatment, and even beyond, patients are constantly asking questions. Through the example of a woman with breast cancer, Strauss and her colleagues showed how the "work" she did was intimately linked to her trajectory as a patient, i.e. to the different phases of the disease she was going through. Before her mastectomy, the authors state that this woman:

> "systematically sought information that would allow her to make intelligent decisions about the next steps. What kinds of operations were possible and feasible? What were the rates of success and failure for each? What were the alternative modes of treatment? What was the reputation of the surgeon to whom she was referred?" [STR 82, p. 981]

To answer these questions, patients can mobilize their relational entourage, composed of lay people and professionals, institutional devices (such as patient associations) as well as digital devices, such as the Internet. The patient is thus considered to have a real health "information system".

Eliot Freidson, with the concept of the lay referral system, highlighted the role played by family and friends in patient information, pointing out that patients did not rely solely on doctors for information and advice about their health [FRE 60]. This attention to the patient's lay environment has subsequently led to a great deal of research that is generally associated with the social support stream. One approach to social support is to describe the individual's social relationships and the resources they are likely to provide. Social resources [LIN 95] are thus considered as assistance, provided by the relational environment, which enables an individual to face a crisis situation [LIN 89], such as the appearance of an illness, by responding to his or her needs. From this point of view, information appears to be a resource that is all the more essential for the patient to whom the pathology generates uncertainty, is a source of anxiety and raises many questions.

However, statistical surveys indicate that 44% of the French used the Internet to obtain health-related information in 2017 (Eurostat data). Given that being ill further accentuates this type of behavior [XIA 14], it is legitimate to ask what place these digital resources occupy in patients' information practices. Recent studies have shown that the Internet is tending to supplant close family and friends and health practitioners as the primary source of information for cancer patients [RUT 16] even though, in terms of trust, the doctor remains the preferred contact [SHE 14]. It is also known that the search for online health information varies according to the socio-economic characteristics of individuals: for example, among cancer patients, studies show that the search for information is positively correlated with the level of education of individuals [CAS 11].

While the production of such statistics relating to the search for information by patients is necessary to understand the phenomenon, it also seems desirable to look at the accounts that individuals give of the steps they take to obtain information and the difficulties they encounter in obtaining this information. This type of approach, which focuses on the experience of the disease, effectively makes it possible to question the reasons behind the information practices of individuals, beyond the quantitative comparisons regularly made between the various available sources.

2.3. Getting information from family and friends when suffering from cancer

2.3.1. *Which relatives are likely to provide what kind of information?*

Among all the contacts present in the patient's entourage, relatives occupy an essential place. They are on the front line, so to speak, in managing the disease in daily life. They give moral support to patients and relieve them, for example, of domestic work that they are no longer able to do. In the context of the generalization of ambulatory cancer treatment, which leads patients to spend more time at home, the role of family and friends is crucial. In addition to material and emotional support, the family and friends of the sick person are also likely to provide the information they are looking for on the disease, treatment or care of cancer. It is therefore common for members of the close circle to seek information from their own side from the moment they learn of the illness affecting their spouse, relative or friend. For these relatives, it may involve consulting the documentation provided by the hospital, consulting the Internet, interviewing their own family and friends, or questioning health professionals. These steps are sometimes taken without the patient's knowledge. But the relatives active in the search for information, if they can communicate useful information, remain nevertheless, in the eyes of the patient, lay people who discover just like him or her the complexity of the cancer pathology and its treatments. In this respect, cancer patients do not expect expert information from these relatives.

Alongside these "neophytes", there may be contacts in the patient's entourage who could be described as insiders. These are friends or family members who have already experienced cancer. These people can then pass on their experience and thus enlighten patients on certain gray areas in the treatment or on the physical or psychological difficulties that await them. These family members or friends who have lived through the cancer experience are interviewed because they themselves have "been there". They are able to provide information that is complementary to that provided by health professionals and of a different nature as it comes from an intimate knowledge of the disease. Patients consider that these insiders provide them with information that is relevant to their personal situation and that they will be able to find a point of comparison to situate themselves in the "world of cancer patients". In addition to the information obtained, the solicitation of this "experienced" entourage effectively allows one to compare one's situation with that of other patients or former patients. Marie Ménoret was able to show how patients carry out a "*situation comparison*" exercise [MEN 07]. With the help of stories of experiences from people around them, patients assess their chances of survival, judge the treatments prescribed to them and confront the side effects they experience.

Finally, the information sought by the patient can be provided by the members of his or her entourage working in the health field. The "doctor friend" or the "nurse sister", for example, is not only likely to directly transmit information about the healthcare system, care and even the course of treatment, but they are, above all, able to mobilize their professional network to obtain information from specialists in the field. It is indeed primarily for their proximity to the medical profession that these relatives can be solicited by patients. Ideally, patients would like to be able to mobilize their oncologist or hospital staff to assist them as soon as they feel the need [DEF 13]. Faced with the difficulties they encounter in soliciting hospital staff, patients may prefer these "second circle" professional sources: if specialists, whom relatives working in the health sector can mobilize through their professional network, do not have precise knowledge of the patient's situation, they have the advantage for the latter of being able to provide information that will be perceived as reliable, scientific and institutional.

Three categories of family members and friends have the possibility of transmitting information of different kinds to the patient: neophyte family members and friends, initiated family members and friends and professional family members and friends. However, not all patients can count on a family and friends who can provide the information they are looking for.

2.3.2. *Difficulty in asking people around you for information*

In general, it is known that the support provided by entourage is unequally distributed among the population. To speak only of the differences in socio-professional categories, a study on self-help (help with moving, financial assistance, etc.) indicates that the average network of helpers for workers is 4.7 people, while the average network of helpers for senior managers is 6.1 people [PET 05]. Cancer patients looking for information are no exception to the rule. However, it is often considered that relatives are a homogeneous group on which individuals can naturally rely in the event of illness. First, there are major differences in the composition of the patient's entourage, generating real disparities between individuals in terms of access to information.

The composition of the patient's entourage varies, first of all, in quantity. It is indeed noticeable that some patients will only be able to rely on a very small number of people to support them during the ordeal they are going through. For some patients, the possibilities of obtaining information from relatives are thus limited, while others benefit from extensive personal networks offering multiple opportunities to obtain information. These disparities in the size of patient networks had already been observed in previous work. Thus, Alexis Ferrand reports the results of a survey conducted by Alexandra Thierry, which shows that women with breast cancer discuss their disease with an average of 13 people in their entourage, but the smallest discussion network observed includes only three people and the largest 31 [FER 11].

Second, the composition of the patient's family and friends varies in quality in the sense that not all the people in the patient's network are likely to provide the resources sought. Some patients will thus be able to mention many relatives working in the health sector, relatives who are active in seeking information or relatives who have themselves experienced cancer. The patients who are most disadvantaged in terms of the composition of their relational entourage will not only have a small number of relatives ready to help them, but these relatives often prove to be "ignorant", just like them, of the cancer treatment modalities, the treatments proposed, the side effects felt, etc. and will therefore not be able to be mobilized by the patients to obtain the information they are looking for. Expectedly, these patients with "unfavorable" entourage most often belong to the most disadvantaged socio-professional categories, such as the 72-year-old breast cancer patient, who had never studied and never worked: during this period, she had only a few relatives in her entourage who supported her, above all, emotionally. And none of these people were able to help her answer the questions she had about her condition and treatments.

Beyond the composition of the entourage, the stories that the patients tell of their search for information also reveal the difficulties they experience in soliciting their relatives and friends, even though some would be able to help them. By integrating this relational dimension, the focus should no longer be on the possibilities offered by the entourage to get information, but on the effective mobilization of relatives as an informational practice. Indeed, while the state of an individual's entourage tells us about the "stock of social resources", it is not sufficient to determine whether these resources are obtained. This non-solicitation of the entourage that we have observed is, first of all, due to a fear of falling into a carer–patient relationship with the relatives. Patients do not want these family and friendship relationships to be governed by medical concerns, such as a patient who refuses to call his or her doctor friend for information about cancer precisely because he or she is a friend. This observation should be seen in the context of patients' desire to distance themselves from being identified as the cancer patient, to which they are constantly referred during their trajectory. In fact, as much as possible, patients stifle their requests to their loved ones so as not to add to the physical stigma they offer to those around them, topics of discussion that "still" concern the disease. In addition, patients will try not to add to the workload that has been weighing on their close relatives since the onset of the cancer. Family and close friends are already under great stress in terms of daily tasks and emotional work to manage the disease. Patients will then seek to use as little as possible these members of their entourage for informational support.

It is also sometimes family members who make the patient understand that they do not wish to be solicited, as some contacts cannot bear to be confronted with the illness of a family member or friend. Without going as far as the extreme position of family and friends who make it clear to the patient that they do not wish to discuss the issue of cancer, patients can get to know their relatives well enough to know whether they have the opportunity, from a relational point of view, to ask them for information about the disease. Thus, the emotional closeness that exists between the patient and his/her love ones limits the possibilities of soliciting contacts that could nevertheless contribute to informing him or her.

Given the difficulties that some patients encounter in obtaining information from their families and friends, digital resources may appear as a means of compensating for this "failure" of social resources.

2.4. Getting information on the Internet when you are sick with cancer

2.4.1. *Widespread use for limited benefits*

It can be seen that the vast majority of patients with an Internet connection at home have used this tool to search for information about their cancer. However, this large proportion of digitally active patients is not sufficient to conclude about the benefits that patients derive from these digital resources. Indeed, it is noted that most patients have difficulty locating the information they are looking for or interpreting it, and that they generally doubt the reliability of the information available on the Internet.

As Paul DiMaggio and his colleagues already pointed out in the 2000s, the inequalities observed between individuals with regard to the Internet are less and less based on access to this technology ("digital divide") and more and more on the ability of individuals to use it efficiently [DIM 04]. For example, some patients simply indicate that they are "not good at it" and see the use of this technology as a real skill to be learned. But even patients who are relatively adept with the Internet tool can have problems finding the health information they are looking for. Beyond technical skills (such as the ability to connect to the Internet or to use a search engine, for example), there are indeed real disparities in terms of information retrieval itself. Patients often do not know the specific terms they should use in their searches or the sites they might visit.

In addition, patients indicate that they are wary of information available on the Internet. While the impressive number of sites and blogs dealing with cancer pathology offers remarkable information opportunities for patients, the way in which individuals view the reliability of the information they find there is a serious obstacle to "digital empowerment", i.e. the emancipatory effect of digital tools, in the sense that they offer individuals more "power to act" [BAC 13]. This lay mistrust is supported by scientific research showing significant differences in the quality of information presented at different sites [FRI 06, HAR 06]. This makes it very difficult for patients to choose between reliable health information and information that may be inaccurate or even dangerous. Individuals point to their lack of medical expertise in this area: ultimately, expert cancer patients are rare. As one patient will say: "To know whether it is reliable or not, you have to be informed already". It is no longer the skills related to the use of the Internet tool that are the problem here but the skills to understand and judge the health information found. Thus, being able to act on one's health, to better manage one's illness by relying on digital tools such as the Internet, does not seem obvious for all patients: it requires specific skills. As noted by Hervé Dumez and Etienne Minvielle who, based on a review of the literature, list the positive effects and risks of e-health in terms of patient engagement:

> "With digital technology, the patient can build up independent expertise. But the quality of this expertise remains fragile. The information may be inaccurate, or require a minimum of professional expertise to be understood" [DUM 17, p. 24].

Similarly, some patients also express concern about finding information that is not relevant to their personal situation. They find it difficult to know whether a statistic or the description of a treatment read on a website, for example, corresponds to their case. When questioning their doctor, patients expect the doctor to take into account their particularities, i.e. both the medical specificities of their pathology and their past history as a patient. Such personalization of information is achieved through the accumulation of patient data. This involves the creation of a medical file, including the medical examinations carried out, the regular recording of vital signs, as well as the repetition of exchanges between the doctor and the patient. Also, it appears much more difficult to obtain personalized information through digital media such as the Internet, compared to the information that can be provided by the oncologist, for example. Even when health websites go beyond cancer generalities, by classifying information according to different situations and by precisely delineating the outlines of this information, patients express their inability to select the information that corresponds to them.

These difficulties that patients encounter in finding information on the Internet are accentuated by the fact that very few patients dare to talk to their oncologist about their search for information. Considering that health personnel in general and doctors in particular are reluctant to this kind of practice, patients anticipate a negative reaction. And when some patients venture to tell their specialist about their Internet use, they feel that their behavior is frowned upon: "If you ask them questions, they tell you 'don't hang around'", says one patient we met. This result confirms a survey indicating that less than 30% of patients who have looked for health information on the Internet say they have discussed it with their doctor [DIA 05]. Relatives can then be invaluable in helping the patient to find information on the Internet. They can guide him or her through the universe of health sites and possibly discuss with him or her the information found. However, this requires that the patient has "connected" contacts in his or her entourage who are enlightened about the pathology and ready to provide support.

Furthermore, given that the median age of patients diagnosed with cancer is over 66 years (according to 2019 data from the French National Cancer Institute) and that the most advanced age groups in the population are known to be less computer-equipped and less connected (according to INSEE data, in 2017, only 42.8% of households over 75 years old are equipped with an

Internet connection), it can be assumed that a significant number of patients do not have an Internet connection at home. If we add this share of "offline patients" to the one we have just described, who have difficulties in exploiting the possibilities offered by the health Internet, we may ask which are the patients who are really able to take advantage of digital resources. We can mention two profiles of "beneficiary patients": patients working in the medical sector, who have the necessary skills to find and sort information, and patients belonging to the wealthiest socio-professional categories. Beyond their ability to search for and interpret information relating to the cancer pathology, these two types of patients are also likely to know, within their family or friendly network, contacts likely to support them in this search for information (e.g. doctors). These remarks are in line with Fabien Granjon's observations on digital inequalities. Beyond the question of access to digital equipment, these also find their source in the ways in which technologies are appropriated and used. Since the capacities to use these tools are socially distributed, digital inequalities must also be seen in the light of the social and cultural capital available to individuals [GRA 12].

2.4.2. *The health Internet: a misleading exposure*

The Internet offers different forms of communication: patients can choose either to consult information only or to participate in discussions by asking questions, formulating answers or reacting to comments [AKR 09]. During our meetings with patients, none of them indicated that they had participated in discussions on forums dedicated to health issues. Although some people admitted to having read the exchanges in which most of the participants were patients or relatives of patients on these forums, what they found there often dissuaded them from going further, like this patient, at ease with the Internet, who explains his reluctance:

> "I've been on these forums.... Every time I've been there, I certainly haven't had any luck because it's a struggle, it's a war […]. I'm less interested, I'm not here to say that".

While the existence of these discussion forums shows that some cancer patients do indeed exchange information about their disease on the forums, it would appear that this type of behavior is not as widespread as their postings would suggest. This observation should not keep us from viewing these numerical exchanges as representative of the behaviors of the entire cancer patient population. When analyzing patient behaviors and opinions solely through the prism of Internet discussions, there is a risk of giving too much weight to the words of individuals who have a digital practice that is not widespread, if not marginal, among the patient population. This figure of the contemporary patient, well described by Eve Bureau and Judith Hermann-Mesfen [BUR 14], also called the connected, informed or even expert patient, has nevertheless managed to impose itself as the standard figure of the patient to such an extent that the question arises as to whether individuals who do not succeed in taking advantage of digital resources do not feel their incompetence in this area as a disadvantageous singularity. The media coverage of the amount of health information available on the Internet and its accessibility, as well as the anxious discourse of the medical profession in the face of this apparent abundance of patient-experts, undoubtedly contribute to reinforcing the feeling, among most cancer patients, that they do not correspond to this figure of the "new patient".

Thus, the "illusion" of the Internet for health and, more generally, digital resources is twofold: first, the extensive use of the Internet to learn about the disease often hides the reality of the benefits that cancer patients derive from it. Indeed, stopping at the number of users of a source of information does not allow us to account for its cognitive effects. Most of the patients we met who used the Internet thus admitted that they were not able to select reliable information and information that corresponded to their personal situation. Furthermore, the posting of cancer patient discussions on the Internet suggests that this is a common practice among the patient population, while it appears that very few patients engage in "online" discussions, based on the interviews conducted during our survey. Thus, the Internet tends to highlight patient opinions and experiences not necessarily found in the offline patient population.

2.5. Conclusion

Regularly seeking to confront digital and social resources leads to dodging/eluding the issue of the difficulties that individuals face in taking advantage of them. However, the accessibility of a resource, in the health field as elsewhere, does not guarantee that it can actually be mobilized by individuals. Thus, rather than opposing these two types of resources, by seeking to determine whether the mobilization of one is to the detriment of the other, it seems necessary to focus on the difficulties that individuals encounter in taking advantage of the digital and social resources available in their environment.

While one might have thought that cancer patients who are disadvantaged in terms of the composition and mobilization of their relational environment would be able to compensate for this lack of social resources with digital resources, it turns out that it is these same patients who face the strongest constraints in terms of obtaining information via the Internet. These patients with cumulative disadvantages often come from the lowest socio-professional categories in the social hierarchy. The discourse on patient empowerment, which heralds the advent of a new, more active, more autonomous and highly connected patient, seems at present to correspond only to a limited fraction of cancer patients, who were already able, long before the development of the Internet for health, to mobilize relational contacts and appropriate mechanisms to obtain information on their disease, such as associative mechanisms to support patients, for example. Thus, by benefiting first and foremost those who need it least, easier access to digital resources would only reinforce the disparities in information among cancer patients.

2.6. References

[AKR 09] Akrich M., Meadel C., "Les échanges entre patients sur l'internet", *La presse médicale*, no. 38, pp. 1484–1493, 2009.

[BAC 13] Bacque M.-H., Biewener C., *L'*Empowerment, *une pratique émancipatrice?,* La Découverte, Paris, 2013.

[BUR 14] Bureau E., Hermann-Mesfen J., "Les patients contemporains face à la démocratie sanitaire", *Anthropologie & Santé*, p. 8, available at: https://journals.openedition.org/anthropologiesante/1342, 2014.

[CAR 14] Cardon D., Smoreda Z., "Réseaux et les mutations de la sociabilité", *Réseaux*, nos 184–185, pp. 161–185, 2014.

[CAS 11] Castleton K., Fong T., Wang-Gillam A. *et al.*, "A survey of Internet utilization among patients with cancer", *Supportive Care in Cancer*, vol. 19, no. 8, pp. 1183–1190, 2011.

[DEF 13] Defossez A., Ducournau P., "Patients receiving ambulatory care: a problematic autonomy situation", *Health Sociology Review*, vol. 22, no. 4, pp. 400–410, 2013.

[DIA 05] DIAZ J.-A., SCIAMANNA C.-N., EVANGELOU E. *et al.*, "Brief report: what types of Internet guidance do patients want from their physicians?", *Journal of General Internal Medicine*, vol. 20, no. 8, pp. 683–685, 2005.

[DIM 04] DIMAGGIO P., HARGITTAI E., CELESTE C. *et al.*, "Digital inequality: from unequal access to differentiated use", in NECKERMAN K. (ed.), *Social Inequality*, Russel Sage Foundation, New York, 2004.

[DUM 17] DUMEZ H., MINVIELLE E., "L'e-santé rend-elle la démocratie sanitaire pleinement performative?", *Systèmes d'Information et Management*, vol. 22, no. 1, pp. 9–37, 2017.

[FER 11] FERRAND A., *Appartenances multiples, opinions plurielles*, Presses universitaires du septentrion, Lille, 2011.

[FRE 60] FREIDSON E., "Client control and medical practice", *The American Journal of Sociology*, vol. 65, no. 4, pp. 374–382, 1960.

[FRI 06] FRIEDMAN D.-B., HOFFMAN-GOETZ L., AROCHA J.-F., "Health literacy and the World Wide Web: comparing the readability of leading incident cancers on the Internet", *Medical Informatics and the Internet in Medicine*, vol. 31, no. 1, pp. 67–87, 2006.

[GRA 12] GRANJON, F., *Reconnaissance et usages d'internet. Une sociologie critique des pratiques de l'informatique connectée*, Presses des Mines, Paris, 2012.

[GRO 11] GROSSETTI M., BARTHE J.-F., CHAUVAC N., "Studying relational chains from narrative material", *Bulletin of Sociological Methodology*, no. 110, pp. 11–25, 2011.

[HAR 06] HARGRAVE D.-R., HARGRAVE U.-A., BOUFFET E., "Quality of health information on the internet in pediatric neuro-oncology", *Neuro-oncology*, vol. 8, no. 2, pp. 175–182, 2006.

[KRA 98] KRAUT R., PATTERSON M., LUNDMARK V. *et al.*, "Internet paradox. A social technology that reduces social involvement and psychological well-being?", *American Psychologist*, no. 53, pp. 1017–1031, 1998.

[LIN 89] LIN N., ENSEL W.-M., "Life stress and health: stressors and resources", *The American Sociological Review*, vol. 54, no. 3, pp. 382–399, 1989.

[LIN 95] LIN N., "Les ressources sociales: une théorie du capital social", *Revue française de sociologie*, vol. 36, no. 4, pp. 685–704, 1995.

[MÉN 07] MENORET M., *Les temps du cancer*, Le bord de l'eau, 2007.

[PET 05] PETITE S., *Les règles de l'entraide. Sociologie d'une pratique sociale*, Presses universitaires de Rennes, 2005.

[RUT 05] RUTTEN L.J.-F., ARORA N.-K., BAKOS A.-D. *et al.*, "Information needs and sources of information among cancer patients: a systematic review of research (1980–2003)", *Patient Education and Counseling*, vol. 57, no. 3, pp. 250–261, 2005.

[RUT 16] RUTTEN L.-J.-F., AGUNWAMBA A.-A., WILSON P. *et al.*, "Cancer-related information deeking among cancer survivors: trends over a decade (2003–2013)", *Journal of Cancer Education*, vol. 31, no. 2, pp. 348–357, 2016.

[SHE 14] SHEA-BUDGELL M.-A., KOSTARAS X., MYHILL K.-P. *et al.*, "Information needs and sources of information for patients during cancer follow-up", *Current Oncology*, vol. 21, no. 4, pp. 165–173, 2014.

[STR 82] STRAUSS A.-L., FAGERHAUGH S., SUCZEK B. *et al.*, "The work of hospitalized patients", *Social Science and Medicine*, vol. 16, no. 9, pp. 977–986, 1982.

[TUB 12] TUBARO P., "Ces réseaux numériques dits sociaux", *Sociologie, Comptes rendus*, available at: http://journals.openedition.org/sociologie/1118, 2012.

[XIA 14] XIAO N., SHARMAN R., RAO H.-R. *et al.*, "Factors influencing online health information search: an empirical analysis of a national cancer-related survey", *Decision Support Systems*, no. 57, pp. 417–427, 2014.

3

Health at the In-between of Computing and the Information and Communication Sciences

3.1. Introduction

The rationalization of medicine and medical organizations began after World War II. It first of all applied to medical decision-making, information production and storage, practice and vocabularies. It then spread to hospital organizations. Since the 1970s, rising health costs have led public authorities to adopt policies concerning the management and regulation of the health system that take precedence over respect for the guarantees of citizens' right to health [OGI 09, CAS 05]. More recently, health informatics plays a central role as an "economic intelligence" tool at the service of public authorities to assist in decision-making and regulation of the healthcare system. If this perspective of health informatics is far from the practice of care in hospitals, it has two major consequences for the development of tools to support the activity. The first consists of incorporating health informatics standards and norms into the technical design; the second is due to the fact that medical information displays a strong disparity between the need for "local" quality linked to the particular management of a patient and the need for "global" quality for the epidemiological, economic and political integration of necessarily standardized information [GRE 09, FIT 13].

Chapter written by Philippe MARRAST.

Health informatics and, more broadly, the standardization of medical or healthcare practices and information with a view to their technical equipment or organizational and managerial support is not a new subject. Whether in the field of decision-making, organization of activity, definition of various nomenclatures, representation of information or even activity support, learning/formalization cycles between norm-required activity and actual and contingent activity have been observed for decades [BER 99, GRO 07].

In this disparity between global rationalization and the organization of daily health activities and the healthcare system, the role of public authorities has become stronger. A major breakthrough occurred in the early 2000s, when the injunction to computerize everything associated with increased financial control and "management" of healthcare activities and health organizations became necessary. Today, the transition to T2A[1], the generalization of ambulatory practice and an aging population are new contextual elements that have led to transformations in the healthcare system, changes in practices and the introduction of new medical standards and regulations.

This renewed context has promoted the emergence of new forms of rationalization of the healthcare system and patient care. Now, the system is moving towards an organizational and technical design centered on the "patient pathway", towards a dematerialization of information and some of the services or support for patients. Thus, the applications of "quantified self", self-monitoring, the numerous online discussion and advice spaces and the rise of remote support (remote consultation, remote prescription, remote support) [MIG 18, OUD 08] have developed strongly [MIG 18, OUD 08].

However, all these innovations, which are sometimes presented as real social, organizational or technical innovations, are associated with increased responsibility and intervention by patients and caregivers. Today, the "good" patient must be an "agile" actor of his or her pathway thanks to "targeted" therapeutic education and support modalities. These are supposed to help develop the skills and support needed to be able to articulate care, therapy, elements for "living well with one's illness", and the various stakeholders in

1 Single mode of financing for the activities of medicine, surgery and obstetrics, both public and private institutions.

this healthcare pathway, which is often made complex in the case of chronic illnesses and comorbidities related to the aging process.

In our research, we question some of the contemporary changes in hospital activity and health in general, linked to the computerization of activities, with a focus on nursing work and more recently on the work of caring for oneself and one's family. In the discourses of the promoters of technologies and new forms of management and in those supporting the various health reforms since 2000, the advent of an automated, "interoperable", "harmonized" and "optimized" environment, populated with machines and software at the service of the different social worlds they equip, is announced. However, in our different fields, we have, above all, observed a variety of relatively heterogeneous or even heteroclite socio-technical assemblages, which only hold together thanks to the efforts of caregivers and patients who work in the creation and translation of information, maintenance and equipment of software, processes and organizations.

In this chapter, we attempt to analyze the way in which the work carried out on social practices in the hospital and research fields has been created and has "developed" us as researchers. In particular, we show how, as computer engineers capable of modeling applications and developing technical functionalities, we are interested in the practices of everyday engineers [VIN 05] who can produce innovations without authors [JEA 07]. These practitioner-generated design objects are valuable sources of information for understanding and analyzing the organization. They shed light on how paradoxical tensions and injunctions are resolved pragmatically [DUJ 08, MIC 11, MOR 09]. They bring ideas to produce a design that is as close as possible to the practice [GRE 09, GRO 07].

We first present the organization in which we conducted our research for three years. We then explain our choices in terms of approach and positioning. We end by developing the theoretical mix that has allowed us to characterize complex organizations.

3.2. The hospital, a field to observe

Within the framework of a research partnership that we have maintained for more than 15 years with a French hospital specializing in cancerology, we have conducted various qualitative studies to address organizational and communication issues. We took interest in the analysis of quality processes, incident reporting, characterization of processes following the computerization of the establishment and the care file[2]. We are currently working with this institution to characterize the transformation of organizational work and to think about social inequalities in health. We are observing patient monitoring devices during chemotherapy treatments and follow-up care, with a focus on the relationship between caregivers and between caregivers and patients.

These different projects were approached in a specific way by a multidisciplinary team and within the framework of an ongoing relationship with the institution. As briefly mentioned in the introduction, public health, because it responds to major societal, financial and organizational challenges, is subject to various rationalizations, standards and regulations of liberal, managerial and/or functionalist inspiration. For Fletcher [FLE 19], understanding the issues at stake in the ramification of the control and management of organizations and professional practices requires research teams to develop multidimensional investigation and analysis strategies and an interdisciplinary approach [OLL 01]. These are the hallmarks of the information and communication sciences.

The different sensitivities and perspectives of successive research teams – built up around management sciences, computer science, sociology, epidemiology, nursing sciences and information and communication sciences – have enabled us to produce over time a kind of scientific heterotopia, specific and contingent. We have thus been able to characterize, over a long period of time, different forms of rationalization of the hospital system as well as the displacement and evolution of certain forms of health professional organizations and practices.

The capacity of this regional hospital specialized in cancerology is about 100 beds. The different services take care of a large number of pathologies and offer various treatments. This establishment recently installed

2 The Electronic Health Record (EHR) is "the written record of all information concerning a patient, which is constantly updated and is used both individually and collectively" [VEN 12, p. 71].

a treatment software, and we were able to observe its integration. Our aim was then to understand some of the changes in the organization of work and the delivery of treatment. More specifically, it was a question of understanding the recomposition of nursing practices during the computerization of the patient record and characterizing the transformation of writing practices following its deployment. Two questions became increasingly acute as the field was visited: how, or through what work, were these complex organizations stabilized? What is this work constituted of to hold together all the heterogeneous elements of which these organizations are made?

After discussion with the nursing staff, we selected three treatment services: day hospitalization, surgery and palliative care. The aim was to represent the variety of care practices and the co-dependencies that exist between the type of pathology, the type of medical acts, the patient management activity and the computer mediation of work. Finally, we also integrated the pharmacy and IT departments. For more than three years, we conducted non-participant observations in the different departments, participated in working meetings and training sessions on the treatment software. These observations were authorized by the healthcare management and under the responsibility of the health executives. In order to "interpret" the organization of work collectives from the environment they inhabit and populate with various objects, we opted for a photo-ethnographic approach [DES 11]. Combined with the techniques of zooming-in, zooming-out [NIC 09] and object biography [BON 15], they allowed us to "see" the organization in multiple micro-, meso- and macro-dimensions, difficult to grasp by simply reading a text or a memo, or through interview techniques. They also gave us the opportunity to "come back" to the interactional scenes and to perceive later in research elements of analysis that had been difficult to understand or detect at the time of observation or in the preliminary analyses.

We also conducted interviews with healthcare management, healthcare executives, nurses, computer engineers and the director of medical information. Finally, we collected technical documents on the technical tools and their infrastructure. In the end, we accumulated more than 100 hours of observations transcribed in four different departments, more than

500 photos, more than 10 hours of videos, more than 20 transcripts of interviews, meetings or training sessions, numerous internal technical documents (hospital information system (HIS) diagrams, specifications of the EHR, EHR user manual, file for reporting “bugs”, EHR paper files).

3.3. An abductive and iterative approach for an “in-between” positioning

The difficulties of being immersed in the research field stemmed as much from the fact that we were discovering a complex environment and that our primary expertise was in the field of engineering and industrial computing, computer science for the Web and telecommunications. Our understanding of the stakes of organizational communication was due, on the one hand, to our experience as a university training manager and, on the other hand, to a resumption of studies in masters in Information-Communication. We therefore had the convictions of an engineer and a self-taught person in the development of techniques that were confronted with a relative lack of reference points in communication. This duality required a great deal of work in terms of translation, adjustment of value registers and acquisition of different concepts and currents of thought.

In a process that ultimately proved to be abductive, the field approach allowed the progressive framing of the object, induced the method and even developed the researcher’s capabilities, at the crossroads between information and communication sciences and computer sciences. The first photo taken on the first day of field work at the hospital (see Figure 3.1) illustrates the socio-technical complexity of medical nursing work that led to our original researcher position. In spite of computer technology, this intern used a variety of documents, means of communication, as well as discussions on the phone or with other caregivers who passed by in the corridor. The identification and then “decoding” of these elements built up expertise in the field [BEC 07] and made it possible to focus on the documentary and more broadly info-communication skills of caregivers [BOU 06].

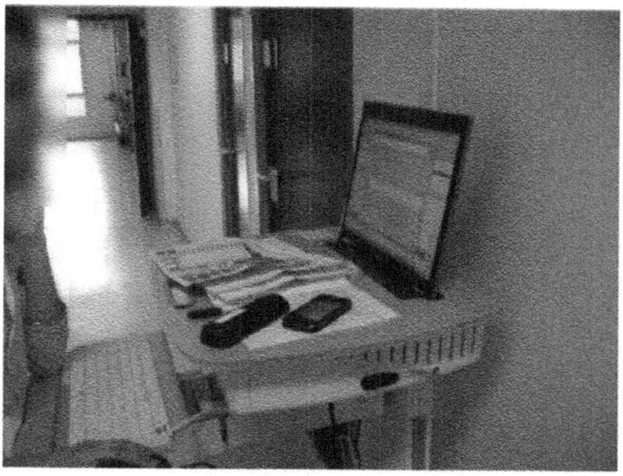

Figure 3.1. *The ecology and socio-technical complexity of medical/nursing work. Variety and heterogeneity of the information material, important work of informational synthesis [MAR 15]. For a color version of the figures in this book see, www.iste.co.uk/morillon/health.zip*

As a counterpoint to these observations, various readings encouraged us to take an interest in the normative network that constrains health informatics. The panoptic of "good practices" for modeling IT applications presented below (see Figure 3.2) illustrates this framing of "concepts" by standards to develop a software architecture and ensure a good level of interoperability for health applications.

We therefore positioned ourselves in this "in-between" of health informatics, combining the points of view of those who developed it as a technical object and those who had to use it on a daily basis, subject to the risks of the care activity. The aim was to understand the diversity of perspectives involved, some of which obeyed to managerial or functionalist heterodoxies and were conceived with a large part of communicational unthought [BOU 08]. But this "in-between" highlights certain epistemological and methodological tensions and even antagonisms between computer sciences that included "modelling, hypothetico-deductive and positivist" and information and communication sciences, generally "interpretative, inductive and constructivist". And it is finally in the course of research that we attempted to propose an open, evolutionary and adaptable computer "model" to various situations of social organizations and to the different modalities of collective actions.

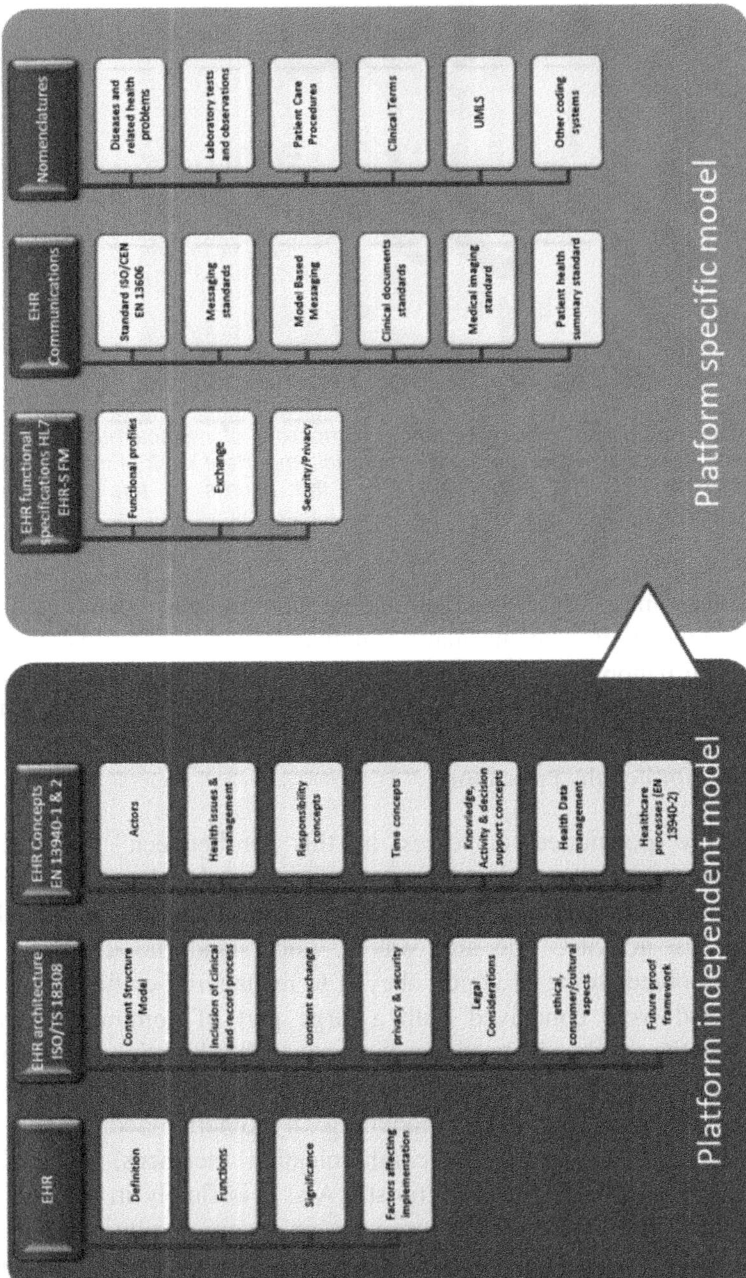

Figure 3.2. *The current set of standards for the design of an EHR [MAR 15]. For a color version of the figures in this book see, www.iste.co.uk/morillon/health.zip*

To do this, we adopted an iterative operation (see Figure 3.3) in order to organize the field survey work; analyzing and coding of this corpus of data; developing the computer model and creating a functional prototype; confronting this theoretical and computer model with the field in order to successively refine the survey work and the robustness of the model and the prototype (which for this purpose was confronted with the evaluation of the actors in the field). Thanks to this abductive and iterative process, rooted in the field, we built up an empirical, situated material that we coded by cross-referencing analyses and readings. We then compared these analyses to the situations on the ground and regularly presented them to the actors. This process allowed us, at each iteration, to gradually withdraw from the contingent and partial nature of our observations and conjectures, to co-construct a robust abstraction of the studied phenomena.

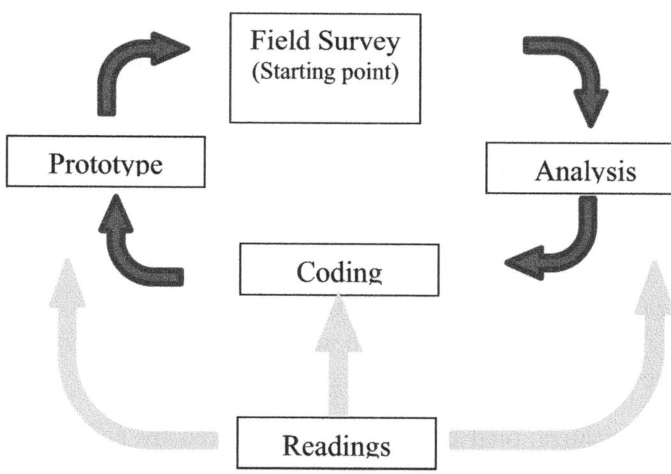

Figure 3.3. *The iterative theorizing process of the embedded theory [MAR 15}. For a color version of the figures in this book see, www.iste.co.uk/morillon/health.zip*

3.4. A theoretical diversity to characterize complex organizations

In order to characterize situations, processes, individual and collective decision-making or organizational and maintenance work in these constrained organizations and complex systems, it must be considered that reductionism and ready-to-think category systems, while powerful tools, can lock the mind into an inadequate framework. Different theoretical frameworks were in fact mobilized.

Technical instrumentalization appeared as a first framework for our reflections. Technology is seen as a socio-technical process with two complementary movements. The first tends to functionalize and standardize our relationship with the world through a traditional technical engineering process. In a second movement, technology is integrated or even hijacked in specific social and technical environments and in the practices and uses of caregivers or patients [FEE 04]. This theoretical starting point and these cross-approaches allowed us to shed light on the issues, the "mechanisms" and the transformative capacities of these organizing technologies. We do not reduce them to their computational characteristics alone. We also included the processes, standards and various formalities of the activity, decision or organization.

We have combined this framework with the method known as grounded theory [GLA 68] according to a constructivist epistemology in the sense of Charmaz [CHA 06]. The latter allows the construction of abstract models of organizations, processes and social phenomena based on qualitative investigations. Oriented towards an objectification of social phenomena, this work is not done "objectively", nor does it "emerge" from theoretical results [GAR 10]. The grounded theories produced are social constructs and the result of iterative and reflexive work [BERT 09], but, above all, situated and contingent and grounded in professional practices [MOR 13]. It is not a question of bringing about a single theory, revealing an essence of social phenomena, but several theories, each adopting different perspectives, paths and therefore different conclusions.

How can organizational complexity, considered by some "rhizomatic"[3] [MEU 13, NIC 09], be accounted for? To do this, we adopted an approach known as "organizational communication". It postulates that communication and communication processes are constitutive of the construction, negotiation, stabilization and continuous adaptation of the organization [TAY 00, LAT 96]. At the same time, the organization – as a recognizable entity – is itself a reference point for carrying out activities, particularly communication activities. Communication and organization are thus continuously co-created, with communication processes and situations drawing the framework of the organization, which is itself the site where

3 Either a heterogeneous network of human and non-human actors who cooperate permanently to stabilize the network, organize and distribute the activity to respond to the contingencies of situations.

communication takes place [STR 92, TAY 00]. In this interweaving, technology plays a special role. Thanks to technical coding, it enables inscribing more or less flexible representations of the organization which help to stabilize processes, roles and structures. Technology also contributes to the activity through powerful presentation, information manipulation and decision support functions. But at the same time, technology is changing the ecology of the activity and can potentially transform the organization, the activity, the modes of coordination and collective action.

3.5. Conclusion

In the thesis that we defended at the end of this work, we were particularly interested in the objects and practices that work on and with the "information system" around the patient record. We were interested in the "sociomaterialities" of work environments [BRU 09, ORL 07, SUC 94], i.e. the way individuals and work collectives "shape" and "update" their environment on a daily basis, as well as the situated ecology of particular objects and practices. We thus considered annotative practices and heuristic writings as organizing and constitutive of the activity [MAR 15]. For example, annotative practice reduces the complexity of the world and hospital activities into micro-fragments of information and stories that can be manipulated by caregivers. The practice of heuristic writing, on the other hand, is a daily and collective work that consists of reassembling the world and the annotation networks in their different facets and dimensions to allow caregivers to feel it, to project themselves into it and to organize and manage future collective action.

We then tried to understand why, despite a rather successful computerization of the patient record, the paper was still very present in the departments, even after several years of using the software. The techniques of multimodal ethnography (audio, video, photo) allowed us to account for the nature of sociomaterialities, their agendas in the activity as well as the dynamics at work in the organizational work that they participate in accomplishing. Among our results, we have, for example, described hybridizations between computer use and handwriting as well as hijacking strategies, engineering writing practices, problem solving, organization and adaptation of activity by caregivers in order to iteratively design a computer prototype. And it is the gaps, the overlapping and "tinkering" that, because they go beyond the strict prescribed framework, allow it to hold. We also found that the accessibility of a resource, in the health field as elsewhere, does not guarantee that it will actually be mobilized by individuals. It then appears necessary to look at the difficulties they encounter in taking advantage of the digital and social resources available in their environment.

In the end, this chapter gives us the opportunity to reflect on the contributions and limitations of our approach and our method for thinking about, on the one hand, the social, technical and organizational dynamics of the healthcare system and, on the other hand, the use of IT equipment in organizations that are more than ever distributed, heterogeneous, dematerialized, global and subject to the pressures of competitive and demanding environments. Our multidimensional and multidisciplinary posture, backed by a qualitative and grounded method, has allowed us to pay attention to the artifacts of the activity, to the design work carried out by the practitioners and to the delicate work of maintaining these artifacts in a dynamic environment.

The "factory" of science as a process encourages us to question the "factory" of the scientist. Thus, while Davallon invites us to think about what "the act of 'constructing' objects in the sciences of info-communication means" [DAV 04], we would in turn call upon a reflection on the construction of the researcher. Doesn't it arise from experiences and interactions with the research object, the field, practitioners or other lecturers? Doesn't the heart of their profession lie in their ability to "think carefully" [PER 17] by allowing themselves this freedom to co-construct and compose with their research objects in order to produce collective knowledge? This is how we see ourselves today as a "hybrid" or even "composite" scientist, combining computer sciences and information and communication sciences to co-construct models with actors in the field.

3.6. References

[BEC 07] BECKER H.P., *Les ficelles du métier: comment conduire sa recherche en sciences sociales*, La Découverte, Paris, 2007.

[BER 99] BERG M., "Patient care information systems and health care work: a sociotechnical approach", *International Journal of Medical Informatics*, vol. 55, no. 2, pp. 87–101, 1999.

[BER 09] BERTUCCI M.-M., "Place de la réflexivité dans les sciences humaines et sociales: quelques jalons", *Cahiers de sociolinguistique*, vol. 14, no. 1, p. 43–55, 2009.

[BON 15] BONNOT T., "La biographie d'objets: Une proposition de synthèse", *Culture & Musées. Muséologie et recherches sur la culture*, no. 25, pp. 165–183, 2015.

[BOU 06] BOUFFARTIGUE P., BOUTEILLER, J., "Jongleuses en blouse blanche. La construction sociale des compétences temporelles chez les infirmières hospitalières", *Temporalités. Revue de sciences sociales et humaines*, no. 4, pp. 39–47, available at: http://journals.openedition.org /temporalites/334, 2006.

[BOU 08] BOUILLON J.-L., "'L'impensé communicationnel'", dans la coordination des activités socio-économiques : Les enjeux des approches communicationnelles des organisations", *Sciences de la société*, no. 74, pp. 65–84, 2008.

[BRU 09] BRUNI A., "Organizational safety: between institutional and sociomaterial practices", *25e EGOS Colloquium*, Barcelona, Spain, vol. 12, pp. 649–678, 2009.

[CAS 05] CASTEL P., DALGALARRONDO P., "Les dimensions politiques de la rationalisation des pratiques médicales", *Sciences sociales et santé*, no. 4, pp. 5–40, 2005.

[CHA 06] CHARMAZ K., *Constructing Grounded Theory: A Practical Guide through Qualitative Analysis*, Pine Forge Press, Newbury Park, CA, 2006.

[DAV 04] DAVALLON J., "Objet concret, objet scientifique, objet de recherche", *Hermès La Revue*, no. 38, pp. 30–37, 2004.

[DES 11] DESALEUX D., LANGUMIER J., MARTINAIS E., "Enquêter sur la fonction publique d'État. Une approche photosociologique des lieux de travail de l'administration", *ethnographiquep.org*, no. 23, available at: https://www.ethnographiques.org/2011/Desaleux-Langumier-Martinais, 2011.

[DUJ 08] DUJARIER M.-A., "Prendre sur soi: l'individualisation du travail d'organisation", in DE TERSSAC G., SAINT-MARTIN C., THEBAULT C. (eds), *La précarité : une relation entre travail, organisation et santé*, Octarès, Toulouse, pp. 107–118, 2008.

[FEE 04] FEENBERG A., *Repenser la technique, vers une technologie démocratique*, La Découverte, Paris, 2004.

[FIT 13] FITZPATRICK G., ELLINGSEN G., "A review of 25 years of CSCW research in healthcare: contributions, challenges and future agendas", *Computer Supported Cooperative Work (CSCW)*, vol. 22, nos 4–6, pp. 609–665, 2013.

[FLE 19] FLETCHER R., "On exactitude in social science: a multidimensional proposal for investigating articulated neoliberalization and its 'alternatives'", *Ephemera, Theory and Politics in Organization*, vol. 19, no. 3, pp. 537–564, 2019.

[GAR 10] GARREAU L., BANDEIRA-DE-MELLO R., "La théorie enracinée en pratique: vers un dépassement de la tension entre scientificité et créativité dans les recherches basées sur la théorie enracinée?", *AIMS 2010*, pp. 1–19, 2010.

[GLA 68] GLASER B.G., STRAUSS A.L., STRUTZEL E., "The discovery of grounded theory; strategies for qualitative research", *Nursing Research*, vol. 17, no. 4, p. 364, 1968.

[GRE 09] GREENHALGH T., POTTS H.W.W., WONG G. *et al.*, "Tensions and paradoxes in electronic patient record research: a systematic literature review using the meta-narrative method", *Milbank Quarterly*, vol. 87, no. 4, pp. 729–788, 2009.

[GRO 07] GROSJEAN S., BONNEVILLE L., "Logiques d'implantation des TIC dans le secteur de la santé", *Revue française de gestion*, vol. 2007, no. 3, pp. 145–157, 2007.

[JEA 07] JEANNERET Y., "Les semblants du papier: l'investissement des objets comme travail de la mémoire sémiotique", *Communication et langages*, vol. 153, no. 1, pp. 79–94, 2007.

[LAT 96] LATOUR B., *Petites leçons de sociologie des sciences*, Le Seuil, Paris, 1996.

[MAR 15] MARRAST P., Equipement informatique des annotations et des pratiques d'écriture professionnelles: une étude ancrée pour l'organisation des soins en cancérologie, PhD thesis, Université Paul Sabatier-Toulouse 3, 2015.

[MEU 13] MEUNIER D., LAMBOTTE F., CHOUKAH, S., "Du bricolage au rhizome: comment rendre compte de l'hétérogénéité de la pratique de recherche scientifique en sciences sociales ?", *Questions de communication*, no. 23, pp. 345–366, 2013.

[MIC 11] MICHAUD V., "Proposition pour l'étude des tensions dans le mouvement, la sociomatérialité et le paradoxe", *Communiquer. Revue de communication sociale et publique*, no. 5, pp. 47–74, 2011.

[MIG 18] MIGNOT P., OMRANE D., "Online info-communication practices in the face of a crisis of trust in breast cancer prevention", in PAGANELLI C. (ed.), *Confidence and Legitimacy in Health Information and Communication*, ISTE Ltd, London and Wiley, New York, pp. 107–134, 2018.

[MOR 09] MORILLON L., BOUZON A., "Les injonctions paradoxales de la communication interne en période de tensions organisationnelles", *Études de communication*, no. 33, pp. 189–202, 2009.

[MOR 13] MORILLON L., BOUZON A., LEE C., "Epistémologies, théories et pratiques professionnelles en communication des organisations", *Études de communication*, no. 40, pp. 9–26, 2013.

[NIC 09] NICOLINI D., "Zooming in and out: studying practices by switching theoretical lenses and trailing connection", *Organization Studies*, vol. 30, no. 12, pp. 1391–1418, 2009.

[OGI 09] OGIEN A., "L'hôpital saisi par la quantification. Une analyse de l'usage gestionnaire de la notion de qualité", *Sciences de la société*, no. 76, pp. 30–51, 2009.

[OLL 01] OLLIVIER B., "Enjeux de l'interdiscipline", *L'Année sociologique*, vol. 51, no. 2, pp. 337–354, 2001.

[ORL 07] ORLIKOWSKI W.J., "Sociomaterial practices: exploring technology at work", *Organization Studies*, vol. 28, no. 9, pp. 1435–1448, 2007.

[OUD 08] OUDSHOORN N., "Diagnosis at a distance: the invisible work of patients and healthcare professionals in cardiac telemonitoring technology", *Sociology of Health & Illness*, vol. 30, no. 2, pp. 272–288, 2008.

[PER 17] PEREZ-BUSTOS T., "Penser avec soin: Effilage et raccommodage dans une ethnographie de broderie artisanale et technologie", *Revue d'anthropologie des connaissances*, vol. 11, no. 1, pp. 1–22, 2017.

[STR 92] STRAUSS A., *La trame de la négociation, Sociologie qualitative et interactionnisme*, L'Harmattan, Paris, 1992.

[SUC 94] SUCHMAN L.A., *Plans and Situated Actions: The Problem of Human-Machine Communication*, Cambridge University Press, Cambridge, 1994.

[TAY 00] TAYLOR J.R., VAN EVERY E.J., *The Emergent Organization: Communication as its Site and Surface*, Lawrence Erlbaum, Mahwah, 2000.

[VEN 12] VENOT A., QUANTIN C., BURGUN A., *Informatique médicale, e-Santé : Fondements et applications*, Springer Verlag, Paris, 2012.

[VIN 05] VINCK D., "Ethnographie d'un laboratoire de recherche technologique: analyse de la médiation entre recherche publique et appropriation privée", *Sciences de la Société*, no. 66, pp. 73–91, 2005.

4

Mental Health and Support for Disaster Victims. Info-communication Devices for Training Volunteer First-aid Workers in a Digital Environment

4.1. Introduction

During a disaster, the psychic impact is experienced in two ways. For individuals, it is potentially traumatic, as those involved may question the meaning of life; for the community, trauma can cause a "crack" in the social fabric, breaking the bond between individuals. Intervening to manage damage, including psychological trauma, is becoming a priority for many researchers who are finding peri-traumatic and post-traumatic disorders (symptoms of mental intrusion, the need to avoid thoughts, places or people related to the event), symptoms of hyperactivity, personality disorders, post-traumatic stress syndromes and post-traumatic stress. In order to reduce these after-effects and facilitate resilience[1], psycho-emotional processes merit being supported (*in situ*), or even monitored (in the long term).

Chapter written by Silvia Rosa SIGALES RUIZ, Erik DE SOIR, Claudia Veronica MARQUEZ GONZALEZ and Michèle CARIA.

1 "The ability of a person or group to develop well, to continue to project themselves into the future despite destabilizing events, difficult living conditions, severe trauma" [MAN 01, p. 17].

In these circumstances, we might expect that the psychological treatment of disaster victims would require specialized training of professional and volunteer rescue and relief teams. Like any training activity, it should be the subject of didactic choices, taking into account established pedagogical principles based on the use of various media. In theoretical terms, the knowledge to be acquired and the skills to be developed would also be based on the work of researchers in this field. In fact, among the sample of existing psychological support measures, the most recent are placed on the Internet because of the generalization of digital tools and their ease of access. What are the contents of these online instruction manuals available to occasional rescuers? On what knowledge bases have they been designed and according to what principles? What is their possible online regulation? Finally, how are acquired skills assessed?

We present here a work carried out within the international scientific network "Environment, Risks and Vulnerability" founded in 2005 by the Universities of Colima (Mexico) and Toulouse (France), which was extended to Belgium in 2006. This interdisciplinary work in the information and communication sciences and disaster psychology began in Mexico with a literature review, mainly on the Internet, and resulted in a qualitative content analysis of eight online instruction manuals available in Latin America. Thus, the aim was to answer the questions previously introduced and also of knowing if these documents met the info-communicational conditions to achieve their objectives. To do so, we present them in detail in their documentary and pedagogical conception as well as in their consideration of the psychological dimensions of mental health and disaster management. After presenting the results, we conclude by inviting questions on knowledge sharing, popularization of science on the Internet and the social involvement of researchers in this context.

4.2. Studying manuals to train volunteer rescue workers in psycho-emotional support for disaster victims

It was only in the 1990s that American researchers studied certain after-effects of the Landers, California (1992) earthquake on a population of firefighters. In the wake of other disasters, the Pan American Health Organization (PAHO) and the World Health Organization (WHO) set the resilience of the affected populations as a goal for responders. Psychological and non-professional volunteers then shared their experiences, but this information was scattered over the Internet. In addition, in most cases, these shared field experiences proposed intervention protocols that were not based on psychological or psychiatric knowledge. Resilience has become such a priority for the member countries of the Hyogo[2] Framework for Action (2005–2015) that PAHO and WHO decided on the direction and organization of psychosocial response to disasters. However, in the field, the large number of disaster victims requiring psychological assistance and the lack of psychologists specialized in the field of post-traumatic stress require the use of occasional first-aid workers, volunteers or general psychologists. In order to help them, some of the disaster responders have therefore freely put online on the Internet feedback on their experience and instruction manuals for the psycho-emotional management of victims and disaster-stricken populations. Therefore, once a lay person (or general psychologist) consults these easily accessible documents, she would think she is "competent" to intervene with disaster victims at the time of first aid.

In order to answer the questions presented in the introduction, in 2015 we produced a comprehensive collection of manuals designed to prepare volunteers for the psycho-emotional support of victims in the event of a disaster [CON 16]. For this purpose, we launched a query on the Internet with the keywords "*intervención psicologica en désastres*" ("psychological intervention in disaster situations"). Fifteen manuals accessible in Latin America and put online between 1999 and 2011 in pdf format were thus listed: four written in English, three of which were incomplete and 11 in Spanish. We finally selected eight manuals in Spanish (see Table 4.5 in the Appendix).

4.3. Four analysis guides

For the analysis, we selected four analysis guides, drawing on Canadian, French, Belgian and Mexican work to explore these documents. We assessed

2 This framework is the main instrument adopted by the Member States of the United Nations to reduce disaster risk. The World Conference on Disaster Reduction spoke out for disaster-resilient nations and communities.

the literature information, instructional design, mental health intervention protocols and disaster management protocols.

4.3.1. *Metadata for online documents*

The metadata[3] recorded in the eight manuals related to the documents and not to the host sites. The analysis was based on the indicators of the 19 Fincowsky criteria [FIN 98] and on the "Quality criteria for electronic publishing sites" selected in the "good practices" of the Maison des Revues site[4]. The following list of metadata summarizes the main documentary features of the manuals:

– none of them offered author profiles, keywords, publication dates, an index, a glossary, a table of contents, the date of online publication, the date of conception or last update;

– none of them indicated a translation in a language other than Spanish;

– two cited the persons responsible for the publication and included illustrations;

– three had logos (Chilean Red Cross, *Centro Nacional de Prevención de Desastres* – CENAPRED in Mexico, Jaume University of Barcelona);

– eight used a title, cited the authors (between two and four for each textbook), offered a summary and paginated the document, indicated the country of preparation, informed that the textbook was free of copyright (copy and print) and specified the file format.

Regarding online navigation and functionalities, the space was structured and the interface prescribed minimum actions in a simple and concise way to access and circulate the document. However, the interfaces were neither ergonomic nor functional: the manuals were simply downloadable text

3 Descriptive elements of the document intended to facilitate access to this document. For online documents: home page, title of the document, language(s) of the text, name of the author, general presentation of the content, keywords, logo, summary, date of publication, date of conception, last update, references and sources, target audience, name of the organization, activity of the organization, place of preparation (country, city), date of publication, etc.

4 Available online at http://www.maisondesrevues.org/327. Working document partially inspired by the quality criteria specified by the Opquast company – http://www.opquast.com/.

documents. Finally, none of the 19 criteria proposed by Fincowsky nor all of the "quality criteria for electronic publishing sites" were met. Therefore, they did not include the expected and necessary metadata for an online educational document.

4.3.2. *Pedagogical engineering of online textbooks*

The analysis of pedagogical engineering was inspired by the ergonomic approach to the design of a training device using the ICT of Tricot and Plégat-Soutjis [TRI 03] and the ADDIE model (Analysis, Design, Development, Implementation, Evaluation) of Basque [BAS 17]. Tables 4.1 and 4.2 summarize, respectively, the pedagogical characteristics of the manuals and the training of designers as well as the resources to which they refer.

The eight manuals offered a general presentation of the content. However, while there was convergence and organization of the concepts addressed, none of them implemented a mechanism adapted to the appropriation of knowledge. They all favored a socio-cognitive model and were based on the idea of learning from a constructivist perspective. The learning, not guided face-to-face by the teacher, was done by the learner [PAT 06]. Yet, the application of such a model remained incomplete because neither the didactic cycle nor the mediation of instructions was planned. Competencies and validation were not announced. There was no provision for learning neither in training units, nor for the possibility of verifying prior knowledge, or of evaluating, after training and in simulation situations, the practical and theoretical knowledge acquired. The textbooks in the corpus did not therefore apply the principles of pedagogical engineering, even though their content explained the conditions that disaster victims may face, possible psychological and emotional behaviors and the psychological techniques to support them. As a result, there was a convergence of the problems addressed, but the gaps in pedagogical engineering did not allow for a rigorous appropriation of information or a validation of skills, due, among other things, to the absence of experts in mental health or disaster psychology.

Issue to be addressed	Expected contents	Presence in manuals
General presentation of the contents (design context)	Purpose: to help the victims psychologically	All
	General objective: to guide volunteers for psychological intervention in a crisis situation	All
	Learners' main objective: to be guided for an intervention	
	Learners' motivations: to intervene, help, rescue psychologically	All
Indication of the profile of the target audience	Any non-specialist wishing to intervene	No prerequisites required
Envisaged learning process	The instructions implicitly lead the learner to transform declarative form knowledge (knowledge) into procedural form (know-how) [AND 00].	The learner will have to produce procedures in real time and in real situations, i.e. use the manual in an unknown context.
Knowledge acquisition	Learning tasks	No exercise is planned, the pedagogical discourse only indicates procedures
	Progress in content	Simple information and technical document
Method of knowledge acquisition	Didactic scenario	None
	Presentation of pedagogical objectives	None
	Regulation of the learner's activity	None
Tutorial	Usage scenario	No indication for the user
Learner follow-up	Interactivity	No interactivity, it is all text to read.
Knowledge assessment	Tests or examination	The manuals only give recommendations at the end of the document.
Evaluation of the device	Control, evaluation, validation	The manuals are freely available online: no validation from a disaster psychology researcher, mental health psychologist, psycho-trauma or post-traumatic stress disorder psychologist.

Table 4.1. *Pedagogical characteristics of textbooks*

Profile of support services	Designer's profile	Designer references
Relief services untrained in psychological response to disasters	No designer is an expert: no mental health psychologist, psycho-traumatic or post-traumatic stress disorder psychologist, no disaster psychology researcher.	– Feedback (three manuals) – Bibliographies in Child Psychology (two textbooks) – References to DSM-IV (four manuals) and various manuals (eight manuals)

Table 4.2. Designer's training and documentary resources

4.3.3. *Mental health intervention protocols*

Content analysis was performed using Tricot's criteria [TRI 03] for content types, Crocq [CRO 87, CRO 99, CRO 07], De Soir [DES 08] and Sigales [SIG 06] for psychological content. Table 4.3 lists the main contents of mental health intervention protocols and whether or not they were taken into account in the textbooks studied.

Most textbooks focused on stress reactions but did not distinguish between normal stress processes (e.g. fear, anger, physiological and psychological reactions, guilt) in everyday situations and normal stress processes in response to abnormal situations (earthquake, flood, terrorist act, etc.) [CRO 87]. All the manuals contained recommendations for crisis intervention, but each presented different techniques. In some cases, however, it was indicated that, after having emotionally relieved the victims, it was necessary to work on resilience. However, this was not defined and no method was proposed. Seven manuals described what a disaster could be; none of them went into detail about the intrapsychic processes that may come into play in a different way for each person. The eight manuals referred to the most recurrent symptoms after impact according to the DSM-IV (Diagnostic and Statistical Manual of Mental Disorders) and to the need to make victims perform an emotional discharge of the lived experience.

Types of content	Expected contents	Presence in manuals
Scope of application	**Disaster situations**	**All**
Objectives	– identify personality alteration – identify the risks of an alteration of the social system – taking into account the traumatic potential of the event – identify psychological processes in direct and indirect (adjacent and/or involved) victims – analyze the victims' predisposition to trauma – identify responses to stress (normal or overwhelming) – identify peritraumatic dissociation reactions – identify cognitive impairments and perceptual functionings – identify prevalence rates of recent somatic, depressive, anxiety and sleep disorders – identify coping strategies dealing with the event – identify dissociative amnesia – identify identity disruption – identify somatoform dissociation – identify physiological reactions	No manual announces these objectives making it possible to understand the immediate psychic reactions with long-term consequences (post-traumatic sequelae).
	– reduce the psychological impact – prevent post-traumatic sequelae – reduce the symptomatology of the repetition syndrome	None of them announces these objectives aimed at reducing post-traumatic sequelae.
	– manage psycho-emotional states – facilitate the expression of feelings and thoughts – raise awareness of the lived experience – facilitate assimilation and integration of the event	The eight manuals announce these psycho-emotional management objectives based on disaster management documentation (WHO and PAHO) or feedback (DSM[5]) or advice from relief agencies.

5 Diagnostic and Statistical Manual of Mental Disorders.

	– promote and strengthen the activation of social networks for social support – provide psychological support – establish the level of intervention by delimiting the action of disaster responders – emotionally stabilize victims – identify victims' stress reactions – provide life safety instructions – build resilience – promote social reorganization – support the return to a normalized situation.	These objectives are aimed at both situational and real-time interventions.
	– develop a briefing and data organization document to provide guidance to victims and their families	A single manual announces this objective for real-time use.
Intervention techniques	– psychological intervention instructions – techniques for calming victims	The eight manuals
Terminology of key concepts	– psycho-emotional reactions – intervention techniques	Identical in all eight manuals
Main activity	– psychological intervention	Four manuals designed by psychologists who do not specialize in first aid support
Knowledge content	– victims' behavioral and emotional reactions – intervention strategies	All these objectives, announced by the manuals, are dealt with
	– contents with reference to the work of experts in post-traumatic sequelae	No reference in the sources of five manuals
Presence of expert committees	– in disaster psychology – in mental health – in post-traumatic stress disorder	No manuals have used experts in these specialties.

Table 4.3. *Main contents of mental health intervention protocols*

In addition presenting a diversity of approaches, the theoretical references in group and crisis psychology were technical and conceptual in textbooks 1,

2, 5, 6 and 7; conceptual from the point of view of developmental and cognitive psychology in textbook 3. In manual no. 4, the theoretical and technical references were based on those of clinical psychology; for the psychosocial dimension; the sources of manual no. 6 were of a technical and conceptual nature; as for manual no. 8, it did not clearly present its theoretical and technical grounding.

For Spanish-speaking countries, the work of the American school, in particular the DSM of the APA (American Psychiatric Association), is currently becoming a model for the assessment, understanding and support of post-traumatic sequelae. However, this approach presents limits to the definition and cataloguing of these symptoms. The broader clinical picture of psychic reactions also becomes more complex. Finally, the contributions of Crocq [CRO 87, CRO 99, CRO 07], De Soir [DES 08] and Sigales [SIG 06] show the psychological stakes in terms of personality, coping strategies, traumatogenic impact and peri-traumatic responses.

4.3.4. *Disaster management protocols*

Content analysis in disaster management is based on the criteria of Crocq [CRO 87], Noto, Huguenard & Larcan [NOT 87] and Contreras, Rosales & Sigales [CON 16]. Table 4.4 presents the main contents of disaster management protocols and their application in manuals.

Five manuals partially addressed the system of disaster management and survival resources provided either by local institutions (*Protection Civile* or fire brigade), by the Ministry of Security or by international actors (Red Cross). Information on the system for the psychological treatment of the population did not appear in any manual; two manuals gave the indications corresponding to the intervention posts of the institutional structures (Red Cross, *Protection Civile*, etc.) as well as their functions and responsibilities. In order to present the affected populations, five manuals described, in an incomplete way, some characteristics of the victims.

Types of content	Expected contents	Presence in manuals
The institutional context	– intervention posts of the institutional structures – coordination and organization of intervention teams – functions and responsibilities of institutional structures – emergency supply management	Five manuals partially
	– information device	No manuals
The population	– classification of categories of persons according to their degree of vulnerability – vulnerability characteristics of the population – definition of types of victims (primary or secondary) – socio-cultural background of the victims	Five manuals partially
The disaster	– disaster classification – disaster characteristics – disaster areas – action priority – identifying the extent of the disaster	Five manuals partially
	– disaster severity levels – cause of disaster – effects in the municipality – duration of the triggering factor	No manuals
The rescue services	– support protocols – organization and coordination of rescue teams – emergency shelter conditions	Eight manuals partially
	– duration of relief efforts – intervention techniques – emergency response plan – identification of evacuation options – casualty management capabilities	No manuals
The information	– the management and operation of accommodation – the region	No manuals

Table 4.4. *Main contents of disaster management protocols*

Four manuals indicated the most important specificities of vulnerability to be identified in relation to children and the elderly. Only three manuals categorized victims (primary/secondary). Two raised the issue of socio-cultural realities (i.e. religion, social organization, etc.). Four manuals offered a classification of disasters and their particularities. Five summarized, in part, the areas of intervention according to the severity of the situation [CRO 87, NOT 87]. All of them addressed the subject of priorities in the intervention and four addressed the scale of the disasters. As for the organization of the relief effort, there was no information on the management or operation of the accommodation for victims.

These manuals are freely available on the Internet for any lay person (or general psychologist) wishing to help victims in disaster situations. As a general rule, it seems that occasional rescuers discover these documents during the event, i.e. when they are applied in real-life situations. It is therefore understandable that they themselves, non-experts, have often neither consulted nor experienced these instructions or advice beforehand. In fact, while the manuals we reviewed provided useful information for describing possible victim behaviors (as per DSM-IV), they did not address the issue of intrapsychic processes. Nor did they give any instructions regarding the respect for the socio-cultural contexts of the victims. However, this psychosocial factor must be taken into account in order to reduce a possible negative influence on resilience when, for example, the population experiences the event as divine punishment [SIG 17]. Similarly, they did not alert to the fact that victims may have normal stress reactions to abnormal situations. If casual rescuers ignore this information, their initial intervention to help may also become a risk factor for victims and another cause of long-term psychological discomfort. Given this observation, how should we design info-communication devices for online training in disaster response?

4.4. An info-communication device for online training in disaster response

For several years now, we have been working on info-communication devices for the prevention and management, particularly psychological, of disasters in France and Mexico. In 2011, we proposed a typology of "info-communication devices at play in disaster reduction" [CAR 11]. We classified these devices into four levels (macro/meso/micro/mini) in their technical, semiological and social dimensions. Today, in order to refine this construction of devices embedded in each other [MEU 99], we propose to define the characteristics of the info-communication devices put on line to support Disaster Response (DICLIC). We conceive them at the meso-level when we study them from the designers' point of view; at the micro-level when we approach them from the perspective of users, occasional first-aiders. Here, we briefly question the info-communication function of DICLICs, distinguishing between primary and secondary devices, and finally define operational mediating devices.

Based on the work carried out in information and communication sciences and in psychology, we believe that DICLICs are affected by several functions insofar as they present interactions and mediations of a socio-technical and semio-technical nature [PER 99]. They also reveal media and enunciative issues [JAC 10, SIM 10] as well as issues of economic, social and political power [APP 10, BER 99, MEY 81]. These devices also engage a pedagogical relationship and, at the semantic level, call for the combination of the three themes to which Lochard refers: intentionality, coherence and uncertainty [LOCH 10]. This theoretical profile now constitutes our "standard meter" for analyzing any DICLIC, taking into account the fact that, for psychologists, the individual, whether designer or user, participates in the device as a subject.

According to Jeanneret, the document includes material characteristics, forms of expression and cultural uses [JEA 05]. The DICLIC, a written document, object or image, socially constructed [COU 09b] by non-specialists, has a humanistic dimension that is supposed to meet the needs of the population. It "exists because [volunteers] need it to prove or explain something" [COU 01 quoted in ENG 09, p. 39]. The document partition is presented in two formats [COU 09a]: the primary device is made up of the media giving direct access to the content (i.e. clinical recommendations, support training); the secondary device is made up of everything that will allow access to the primary device (online electronic documents). However, the nature of the link that may exist between physical places, people, standards, languages, common know-how [FRA 09] needs to be specified.

The DICLICs disseminated online by the designers – facilitators of the dissemination and circulation of information [FRA 09] relating to first aid – are documents intended, on the one hand, to inform the general public on the attitudes to be adopted or banned. On the other hand, they are used to train in the know-how and skills experienced in the field, reformulated and explained on the basis of the feedback presented or received. This observation leads us to define the conditions for building knowledge, sharing it and applying it in the field. Designing such mediating devices, freely accessible on the Internet, in an educational perspective and based on the instructions contained in official documents, requires associating designers and researchers, experts in disaster psychology and educators, in order to develop a knowledge to be communicated and communicable [MEY 86]. In other words, a mediating device, in this case a meso-dispositive one, must allow a social and shared learning of disaster intervention and management by taking into account the dimensions of socio-technical and semio-technical orders [PER 99] as well as the three Lochard themes [LOC 10].

4.5. Conclusion

In the context of a disaster, treating the psychological impact becomes as much a priority as saving lives. The mental health risks that lead to psychotrauma include the development of other long-term psychopathological, psychosomatic and even psychosocial health problems in the victim population. In this context, while the Internet can be a useful resource for coping, the ease with which documents can be deposited on it and then made freely accessible invites researchers to initiate different types of reflection: theoretical in mental health psychology in the context of disasters, ethical, epistemological in terms of implexity and, finally, deontological in order to "protect the public from the misuse of psychology and the use of methods and techniques abusively claiming to be psychological"[6].

Thus, the manuals in our corpus, all accessible on the Internet, were designed on the basis of "feedback from experience", a methodology specific to the field of emergencies in Europe, particularly in the context of disasters. They were not DICLICs because they did not meet all the pedagogical conditions of a training system and were not based on the theoretical and deontological foundations of psychology. It would seem that we are therefore in one of the four communication situations proposed by Véron [VER 97]: exogenous communication about science, since the designers publish their know-how for the general public without knowledge

6 (French) Code of Ethics for Psychologists (1996, updated in 2012). http://www.codededeontologiedespsychologues.fr/LE-CODE.html.

of the field they are dealing with (the psychology of psychological trauma in emergency situations), nor of the methods for teaching it (pedagogy and didactics). This lack of specific methodology in terms of support exposes victims to additional risks. In the field of health, the Internet could weaken the status of expertise, or even the legitimacy of a scientific field, as emergency psychology could be considered as a "pseudo-science".

Under these conditions, preserving the scientific validity of knowledge disseminated on the Internet to deal with sensitive situations such as mental health may encourage the researcher to intervene through applied research, action research and/or popularization. Moreover – using Veron's categories [VER 97] – the development of endogenous intra-disciplinary communications (between researchers in psychology) and endogenous inter-disciplinary communications (between researchers in psychology and researchers in pedagogy, experts in the design of online devices) appears more essential than ever.

4.6. Appendix

Manual Code	Website	Name of the manual	Place and Year
APSCFNN05A-2011-CHL 1	http://www.crececontigo.gob.cl/wp-content/uploads/2010/07/Apoyo-Psicol%C3%B3gico-en-Situaciones-de-Crisis-para-Familias-con-ni%C3%B1os-y-ni%C3%B1as-de-0-a-5-a%C3%B1os.pdf	Apoyo psicológico en situaciones de crisis para familias con niños y niñas de 0 a 5 años: Orientaciones técnicas para equipos de salud, educación inicial y voluntariado.	Chile 2011
PPSE-2011-MX 2	http://sismos.gob.mx/work/models/sismos/Resource/68/1/images/atencion.pdf	Preparación Psicológica en Situaciones de Emergencia.	Mexico 2011
APIDDEEP-2010-ESP 3	http://repositori.uji.es/xmlui/bitstream/handle/10234/79707/forum_2001_13.pdf?sequence=1	Análisis de un programa de intervención en desastres dirigido a estudiantes de educación primaria.	Spain 2010

ICSD:IPSI-2009-CR 4	http://www.binasss.sa.cr/revistas/rmcc/587/art1.pdf	Intervención en crisis en situaciones de desastre: intervención de primera y de segunda instancia (revisión bibliográfica).	Costa Rica 2009
IPSED:GPAP-2007-CHL 5	http://diversidad.murciaeduca.es/orientamur2/gestion/documentos/2-intervencion_psicosocial.pdf	Intervención psicosocial en situaciones de emergencias: guía del primer apoyo psicológico.	Chile 2007
IPSED-2004-ESP 6	http://www.ipbscordoba.es/uploads/Documentos/Publicaciones_Ipbs/Protocolo_ipcased.pdf	Intervención Psicológica ante Situaciones de Emergencias y Desastres.	Spain 2004
MICSD-2001-SV 7	http://www.psicosocial.net/grupo-accion-comunitaria/centro-de-documentacion-gac/areas-y-poblaciones-especificas-de-trabajo/carceles/3-manual-de-intervencion-en-crisis-en-situaciones-de-desastre/file	Manual de Intervención en Crisis en Situaciones de Desastre.	El Salvador 2001
RP:UGFACD-1999-COL 8	http://www.amauta-international.com/Trauma.pdf	Recuperación Psicosocial: Una Guía para Facilitadores de Apoyo en Crisis y Desastres.	Colombia 1999

Table 4.5. *Abbreviations and coding of the Spanish textbooks available on the Internet and selected for the study*

4.7. References

[AND 00] ANDERSON J.R., *Learning and Memory, an Integrated View*, 2nd ed., Wiley, New York, 2000.

[BAS 17] BASQUE J., Introduction à l'ingénierie pédagogique, 4th ed., Cours en ligne TED 6312 Ingénierie pédagogique et technologies éducatives, Université TÉLUQ, Montreal, Canada [Online]. Available: http://ted6313v2.teluq.ca/teluqDownload.php?file=2014/04/19_TED6313_Texte_Intro_IP.pdf, 2017.

[BER 99] BERTEN A., "Dispositif, médiations, créativité: Petite généalogie", *Hermès La Revue*, no. 25, pp. 33–46, 1999.

[CAR 11] CARIA M., SIGALES RUIZ S., AGUIRRE Z. *et al.*, "Prévention des catastrophes et dispositifs info-communicationnels: une collaboration scientifique interculturelle", in COUZINET V., COURBIERES C. (eds), *Médiations et hybridations: Construction sociale des savoirs et de l'information, actes du 2ème colloque scientifique international du réseau MUSSI*, Toulouse, France, pp. 187–199, 2011.

[CON 16] CONTRERAS-PEÑA V., ROSALES-CHAPULA D., Análisis documental de los programas y/o protocolos de intervención psicológica en situaciones de desastres, Thesis, SIGALES RUIZ S. (ed.), Universidad de Colima, Mexico, 2016.

[COU 01] COUZINET V., REGIMBEAU G., COURBIERES C., "Sur le document: notion, travaux et proposition", *Jean Meyriat, théoricien et praticien de l'information-documentation*, ADBS Éditions, Paris, pp. 467–508, 2001.

[COU 09a] COUZINET V., *Dispositifs info-communicationnels: contributions à une définition. Dispositifs info-communicationnels: questions de médiation documentaire*, Hermès-Lavoisier, Paris, pp. 6–17, 2009.

[COU 09b] COUZINET V., "Complexité et document: l'hybridation des médiations dans les zones en rupture", *RECIIS Electronic Journal of Communication Information and Innovation in Health*, vol. 3, no. 3, pp. 10–16, 2009.

[CRO 87] CROCQ L., DOUTHEAU C., SAILHAN M., "Les réactions émotionnelles dans les catastrophes", *Encyclopédie Médico-Chirurgicale-Psychiatrie*, 37113 D, pp. 2–8, 1987.

[CRO 99] CROCQ L., *Les traumatismes psychiques de guerre*, Odile Jacob, Paris, 1999.

[CRO 07] CROCQ L., *Traumatismes psychiques*, Masson, Paris, 2007.

[DES 08] DE SOIR E., ZECH E., VERSPOTEN A. *et al.*, "Prédiction de l'ESPT lors d'une catastrophe technologique (Ghislenghien, 30 juillet 2004)", *Stress et Trauma*, vol. 8, no. 3, pp. 211–224, 2008.

[FIN 98] FINCOWSKY-FRANKLIN E., *Organización de Empresas: Análisis, diseño y estructura*, McGraw-Hill Interamericana, Mexico, 1998.

[FRA 09] FRAYSSE P., "Outils, documentation et ressources pédagogiques: un dispositif info-communicationnel de l'éducation, le SCEREN", *Dispositifs info-communicationnels: questions de médiation documentaire*, Hermès-Lavoisier, Paris, pp. 33–70, 2009.

[JAC 10] JACQUEMIN B., "Un dispositif de collaboration: l'exemple de Wikipédia", in APPEL V., BOULANGER H., MASSOU L. (eds), *Les dispositifs d'information et de communication. Concept, usages et objets Collection Culture & Communication*, De Boeck Supérieur, Brussels, pp. 117–136, 2010.

[JEA 05] JEANNERET Y., “Dispositif”, in SOURY C. (ed.), *La “Société de l’information”: glossaire critique*, Commission Nationale Française pour l’Unesco, La Documentation française, Paris, pp. 50–51, 2005.

[LOC 10] LOCHARD G., “Une approche sémantique du dispositif: l’exemple des événements sportifs à la télévision”, in APPEL V., BOULANGER H., MASSOU L. (eds), *Les dispositifs d’information et de communication. Concept, usages et objets*, De Boeck Supérieur, Brussels, pp. 187–199, 2010.

[MAN 01] MANCIAUX M. (ed.), *La résilience : résister et se construire*, Médecine et Hygiène, Geneva, 2001.

[MEU 99] MEUNIER J., “Dispositif et théories de la communication”, *Hermès La Revue*, no. 25, pp. 83–91, 1999.

[MEY 81] MEYRIAT J., “Document, documentation, documentologie”, *Schéma et schématisation*, no. 14, pp. 51–63, 1981.

[MEY 86] MEYRIAT J., “La science de l’information”, *Revue des sciences morales et politiques*, no. 2, pp. 255–269, 1986.

[NOT 87] NOTO R., HUGUENARD P., LARCAN A., *Médecine de catastrophes*, Masson, Paris, 1987.

[PAT 06] PATINO M., “Modelo socio-cognitivo: Teoría educativa y de diseño curricular”, *Medicina Interna, Educación Médica y Comunidad*, vol. 22, no. 1, pp. 17–40, 2006.

[PER 99] PERAYA D., “Médiation et médiatisation: le campus virtuel”, *Hermès*, no. 25, pp. 153–167, 1999.

[SIG 06] SIGALES-RUIZ S., “Evaluación Longitudinal sobre los Estados postraumáticos vinculados a las catástrofes industriales. El caso de la población de San Juan Ixhuatepec (México)”, *Anales de Psicología,* vol. 22, no. 1, pp. 22–28, 2006.

[SIG 17] SIGALES-RUIZ S., CARIA M., “Los desastres en México de los 80’s: Miedo, culpa y secuelas psicosociales”, *Les Cahiers ALHIM*, no. 34, pp. 22–28, 2017.

[SIM 10] SIMMONOT B., “Les moteurs commerciaux comme dispositifs d’accès à l’information en ligne”, in APPEL V., BOULANGER H., MASSOU L. (eds), *Les dispositifs d’information et de communication. Concept, usages et objets*, De Boeck Supérieur, Brussels, pp. 95–115, 2010.

[TRI 03] TRICOT A., PLEGAT-SOUTJIS F., "Pour une approche ergonomique de la conception d'un dispositif de formation à distance utilisant les TIC", *Sciences et Technologies de l'Information et de la Communication pour l'Éducation et la Formation*, vol. 10, pp. 217–254, 2003.

[VER 97] VERON E., "Entre l'épistémologie et la communication", *Hermès La Revue*, no. 21, pp. 25–32, 1997.

PART 2

Thinking about the Ethics of Health Research in a Digital Context

5

Ethical Positions Arising from Research on Online Communities in the Health Sector

5.1. Introduction

A qualitative research project in the information and communication sciences (ICS), questioning the new digital mediations of health knowledge and the digitalization of social support between patients and/or carers, led to the observation of communities in the online health sector. This research project, funded as part of the LipSTIC Laboratory of Excellence, which aims to combat cancer and inflammatory diseases through the use of lipoproteins as nanovectors, investigated interactions in online discussion and information exchange spaces focused on health and, in particular, cancer and chronic diseases. This research has mobilized empirical approaches based mainly on ethnographic observation methods, involving the use of experiential, sometimes very personal, statements that require caution and precautions regarding respect for the testimonies collected and the integrity of the respondents.

From the outset, our research position was questioned, both individually and collectively. The specificity of the fields, our possible interaction with community members, the context underpinned by an evolving legislative

---

Chapter written by Aurélie POURREZ, Elodie CRESPEL, Stéphane DJAHANCHAHI, Olivier GALIBERT and Benoît CORDELIER.

framework,[1] the methodological choice of data collection and the research themes imposed on us the need to put the ethical issues into perspective. We can now consider this question at least on three levels. The first concerns the classic caution of any social scientist in the face of the testimonies collected and analyzed. It is a question of not betraying the purpose of the survey, while possibly respecting the anonymity of the respondent in order to protect him or her. At a second level, cautious and distant action is at the heart of ICS research, which proposes an analytical framework for traces of online interactions. The interviewer can then choose to be identified as a researcher by the online observed community, without the interviewee having explicitly agreed to be an observed subject. From this point of view, it seems that the human and social sciences (HSS) did not follow the explanatory recommendations to participants before collecting their consent before the Jardé Act [VAS 08]. Although France has not integrated this search for consent into its practices, the United States was been obliged to do so since 1981, Canada since 1998 and England since 2005. At a third level, there is the question of observations of info-communication practices in a digital context, the purpose of which is the mediation of knowledge and social support in health. Indeed, this field of activity, which is highly regulated, implies that the user member of an online community dedicated to intimate information must make it visible.

At a time of massive exploitation of public and private data on the Internet (big data) and a public desire for legal regulation (GDPR[2]), the question of the ethical stakes of health research in ICS appears to us to be central and is the subject of this chapter. To do this, we first categorize scientific ethics in empirical and methodological practices. Next, we present the empirical, ethical and methodological info-communication issues raised by our research program in digital technologies, information, communication (DIC) and health, marked mainly by ethnographic approaches.

1 The Jardé Law, No. 2012-300 of March 05, 2012, sets out the general principles relating to research involving the human person. It was originally intended to apply to all disciplines. Given the scope of the protocols to be submitted, an ordinance in June 2016 and an implementing decree in November 2016 excluded HSS research from the scope of the law.

2 The entry into force on May 25, 2018, subsequent to our research, of the General Data Protection Regulation (GDPR – No. 2016/679 of the European Union), repealing Directive 95/46/EC, did not constrain our handling and regulatory compliance of the data obtained.

5.2. Epistemology, deontology and ethical reflection

In this first part, we attempt to address the construction of the ethical question for the ICS researcher questioning socio-technical info-communication devices in health. In order to do this, we, first of all, propose an argument on the need for ethical questioning as an element of scientific reflexivity. Next, we consider the relevant elements of an empirical and methodological ethics of research conducted on the uses of NICTs. Finally, we outline empirical and methodological ethics for the understanding of digital mediations in health.

5.2.1. *From the necessary scientific reflexivity to empirical and methodological scientific ethics*

The specificity of ethical reflection in qualitative health research [FOU 16] stems from the interaction between the field, the subjects studied and the researchers [CAR 04]. The co-presence of researchers and subjects, the relational quality thus established and the consideration of the representations of all the actors co-construct in part the commitment and the scientific production. The establishment of professional rules allows for the implementation of a research protocol, but does not ensure a constant reflexivity as to the posture adopted. It is therefore necessary to go beyond a mastery of scientific routines (theoretical basis, ability to problematize, development of a methodology, etc.) in order to question the exercise of research in a normative way.

Beyond an institutionalized or tacit professional regulation, implementing a scientific approach implies the subjective as well as intersubjective mobilization of scientific ethics. The latter constitutes a significant part of the researcher's professional identity and professionalism [BOU 91]. Beyond the elements related to recognition and peer review or the risks of instrumentalization of the results produced, to which we shall return at the end of this chapter, the methods of data collection and the limits imposed on the researcher during this collection concentrate a good part of the ethical precautions of the researcher in the HSS and, *a fortiori*, in CIS. The "sanitary" nature of the data collected for those interested in the field of health and care adds an extra level of attention. Indeed, the vulnerability of the interviewees, fueled by a serious pathology, immediately calls into question our responsibility. This context, which can be described as morbid, accentuates an asymmetry in the investigator/investigated relationship, which is denounced through the power and authority of the researcher [BAL 93].

Three types of reflexivity can be classically envisaged: personal (as mentioned above), functional (putting in tension an appropriation of professional rules and values) and disciplinary, as they are expressed at the institutional, social or political levels [WIL 88]. However, this scientific commitment and willingness to adopt a rigorous approach is not an ethical stance in itself. Nevertheless, reflection is present in the scientific approach in HSS, from the determination and negotiation of an epistemological posture.

Morality, indicible but underpinned by injunctions to ethics, has a double function: on the one hand, "the region of norms, the principles of permissibility and prohibition" and, on the other hand, "the feeling of obligation as the subjective face of a subject's relationship to norms" [RIC 04, p. 689]. Ethics here is situated on both sides of these norms: upstream and downstream of moral norms. In this sense, Ricoeur calls for a practical wisdom for which we cannot pre-establish ethical rules to be respected. Thus, a concern with the ethical issue of research does not constitute the establishment of rules or standards. It is a reflexivity put in tension by practice. It is the field, the interactions between its actors that will impose a research posture imbued with this practical wisdom. The work of preparing the research protocol aims at identifying, making visible and anticipating the elements that may call for a confrontation with the standards. Through its analysis, the digital context invites research practices to take into account traceability, visibility and the possible diversion of observed uses.

5.2.2. *ICS and methodological and empirical ethics related to the study of NICTs*

Beyond an epistemological and methodological definition that may be either singular to each specificity established by this interdisciplinarity or crossed in the community of ICS researchers, the constructed info-communication research objects sketch a complex empirical environment. This is notably due to the fact that the ICS are identified for their expertise in the analysis of socio-technical communication devices

(Community Services and Applications on the Internet [GAL 14]). Today, the Internet is the space for all the controversies in health as well as for all the hopes of economic, political or associative actors concerning the accompaniment or information of patients and caregivers. The ICS community, which is very active in the field of health, is therefore at the heart of empirical and methodological issues at the confluence of precautions related to the possibilities of massively collecting personal, potentially intimate data, whether on public expression spaces (e.g. discussion forums, Facebook pages with unrestricted access, influencer's Instagram account) or closed (e.g. online communities whose access must be validated by the administrator).

Nevertheless, like all the HSS, the ICS does not have an ethical guideline that would institutionalize the researcher's ethics. For professional bodies that have one, it is a set of duties related to the practice of a profession, based on shared practice and values. These are legal rules that reflect moral standards and for which sanctions are imposed for non-compliance (where non-compliance with moral standards is limited to the examination of conscience and/or disapproval [SIR 04]). Just because there is no ethical guidelines does not mean that the ICS researcher's position is unethical. It must therefore work within the framework of "good practices" involving attitudes, behavior, procedures and different levels of responsibility (institutional, professional and personal). The ethical concern should therefore not leave him/her during the protocol, neither upstream nor during the exploitation of the data. This concern is all the more necessary in the context of research attempting to identify, analyze and understand the uses and practices of socio-technical info-communication devices.

Indeed, the studies we conducted were partly based on traces left online by patients or their relatives. The HSS web analysis manual published by Barats [BAR 13] offers a panorama of web approaches. Although data published on the Internet are unknown to their authors who may remain unknown, data collected online cannot be called public. As the authors remind us, what is private may become public, what is public may have been enunciated within a framework that is felt to be private:

> "Each social context has its own system of norms (often implicit) governing the types of information that it is appropriate to share with others and redistribute to third parties. When these standards are violated, it is important to become

> familiar with these 'informational standards', which are part of the local norms governing online interaction spaces known as 'netiquette'" [BAR 13, p. 48].

On the one hand, this implies that the researcher must be sensitive to anything that may be harmful to individuals and "...not take for granted such common notions as public/private distinction, anonymity or consent" [BAR 13, p. 48]. On the other hand, these local standards are part of a set of methods and processes of exchange, creation of specific codes, construction of meaning and organization of communities. "These methods that members use in their social activity" [LAH 92, p.81] are studied by ethnomethodology [GAR 67, COU 14].

5.2.3. *Empirical and methodological ethics*

For HSS, anthropologists first established principles of responsibility. Health ethics, particularly in clinical experimentation, is essentially concerned with respect for principles and the protection of persons (the benefit/risk ratio is only studied if ethical principles are respected). Uncontrolled clinical experimentation in medicine continued beyond World War II and was repeated until the Tuskegee scandal, in which the African American population in a region of the United States was subjected to experimentation to improve knowledge about the natural course of syphilis when a treatment was available. This research has lasted more than 70 years. When the scandal broke, principles were laid down[3] (autonomy, beneficence, *primum non nocere*[4] and justice) to prevent the possibility of such practices. In HSS, the survey on homosexual encounters in public toilets [HUM 61] or the survey on authority and obedience [MIL 63] and others led to the creation of the American Anthropological Association and the American Sociological Association, whose principles are based on those of clinical research actors: respect, beneficence and justice [FOU 16].

3 The Belmont Report, established in 1979 following the denunciation of the scandal, led to the development of bioethical principles in the United States. Failure to respect these principles, even today, leads to the inadmissibility of a study and its results far beyond the United States.

4 "first do no harm".

In the United States, universities have gradually set up ethics committees to monitor certain aspects of research carried out by their researchers. These committees were set up for biomedical research in 1974, and then extended their activity to HSS research since 1981. Canada and then England, as well as Switzerland and other European countries, impose the same obligation on HSS researchers. In France, many universities, as well as some HSS laboratories (e.g. the CRFPD Psychology Laboratory at the University of Rouen), have set up ethics committees, albeit with an advisory role.

The texts that frame the ethical procedures of Canadian universities are based on three guiding principles: respect for people, concern for welfare and justice. These texts can easily serve as a first reading for beginners and even more experienced researchers when faced with new issues related to their fields. They are particularly relevant to establishing the decision-making capacity of groups of individuals to consent before participating in research, understanding the ethical implications of privacy and confidentiality, potential conflicts of interest, concern for the welfare of participants or determining the anticipated level of risk to research participants.

The ethical issues related to research on online health communities were formulated, for example, by Christine Thoër [THO 12], following the work of Christine Hine [HIN 05]: (1) access to online exchanges, (2) whether or not it is necessary to obtain consent from participants, (3) the procedures for contacting participants and obtaining free and informed consent, (4) managing the risks associated with participation in the research project, which are all the more greater as the issues under study are sensitive and (5) the presentation and dissemination of research results. Based on this, we discussed some positions taken in netnography: is it necessary to identify oneself as a researcher or to pretend to be a user in order to access exchanges? Since the French law did not oblige us to do so, was there a need to, beyond guaranteeing respect for anonymity, collect the consent of the participants, particularly in the context of ethnographic observations, by presenting the research protocol to them more precisely? In the subsequent section, through the actions we put in place in the collective research project on online health communities, we will try to provide practical answers to these questions.

5.3. Empirical and methodological ethics in ICS and digital health

The actions that, in our view, reflect the application of an empirical and methodological ethics in our ethnographic approaches focus on the following three questions: is it necessary to obtain explicit permission from the interviewees to observe and analyze the digital traces of their interactions? Does the researcher-observer have to reveal himself or herself to his or her observers? How can we protect both the observed user members and the researcher-observers?

5.3.1. *Collecting authorizations and approvals*

As part of our empirical approach, we designed a file to be submitted to the Comité de Protection des Personnes, CPP (French Committee for the Protection of Persons). At the same time, a new decree implementing the Jardé law was under discussion, as the CPPs could not assume responsibility for the study of all clinical and HSS research. The file consisted of the research protocol, a summary of the protocol, a list of investigators, an information letter to the people included in the protocol and a consent to collect. The Directorate General of Health, to whom we addressed ourselves at the request of the CPP in order to obtain details on the procedure to be followed for our protocol, replied to us after receiving our file:

> "The project does not aim to develop biological or medical knowledge, and therefore does not fall within the scope of research involving the human person. Rather, as your subject indicates, it is research in the field of information and communication sciences. It does consist of interviews with patients, but this is a health survey, and if health data is collected from individuals, it is in the opinion of the CNIL. The opinion of a CPP is therefore not required".

Not seeking to collect health data from individuals, neither the CNIL nor the CPP could assure us of compliance with the principles that we could only assume. As the decree implementing the Jardé law was imminent, we requested the scientific referent of the university house without obtaining any guarantee on the respect of the legislative framework. Moreover, when we presented our results, the forthcoming entry into force of the GDPR threatened our presentations with not being in line with it. This concern to respect the legislative framework questioned our practices and customs, but did not constitute an ethical approach. We have therefore mobilized an unspoken ethical guidelines and legislation in the making to determine our professional stance.

Once the selected sites had been distributed[5] among the project researchers, it was only through consultation that we were able to establish the ethical issues beforehand. The topics of discussion concerned cancer, its experience, its treatments prescribed by the medical profession or suggested by alternative practices. The subjects to be observed had a health or emotional state that indicated vulnerability. Much more than making explicit a current concern that was essential for obtaining funding or publication (submission to an ethics committee), establishing the postural ethical implications was necessary for the methodological choices and their implementation in the field [FOU 16]. For example, what information should be given to the "owner" of the Service and/or the Community Internet Application (SACI) or to the Community Manager? Did our research have to be visible and thus take the risk of being denied access to the field? Or do we choose to pretend to be a member of the community without implying that we are conducting research? In the section below, we will try to enrich this question, which is peculiar to many research projects based on online ethnographic approaches, with our experience.

5.3.2. *Concealing or revealing oneself as a "researcher-observer"?*

For the field www.lesImpatientes.com, the decision was taken to pass the file constituted for the CPP by adapting it to the forum moderators. This community site is for women affected by breast cancer. Here, information can be found on treatment modalities, side effects, the experiences of others, solidarity in the face of the disease, the treatments induced and the consequences on daily life, especially family life. A forum by themes is readable by all, and registration is necessary to participate. Observation having made us doubt the topicality of their activity and having no feedback, we opened an account not to participate in the forum, but to access the directory and email addresses of the Impatientes. So it was by email that we solicited them by introducing ourselves and explaining the objective of the research, explaining that we did not want to interfere in the

5 www.Doctissimo.fr; www.lesImpatientes.com; www.cannaweed.com/forums.

discussions, that we wanted to conduct an interview and that without feedback from them, we would not insist. We thus obtained answers and exchanged and even carried out telephone interviews. Without introducing ourselves, we could have exchanged directly by email with a larger number of Impatientes, but pretending to be a person suffering from cancer and asking for solidarity to achieve this was of course not an option.

In this way, we could directly link the ethical issue and the methodological construction of the protocol based on the principle of primum non nocere. Since the exchanges took place at the time of a live experience of the disease during which the person developed defense mechanisms, to what extent did our intervention not interfere in the development of these strategies? For the Impatientes, we endeavored to make the volunteers feel comfortable about the freedom of their participation and committed to a caring and humble attitude. In response to the discourses we came across, previous reflexes of active listening by a caregiver were mobilized, as well as the clinical knowledge of a researcher on the team, who had a professional background as a nurse. Humility consisted of differentiating ourselves from a caring relationship and, above all, not to interfere with the latter. Indeed, could our investigation harm a psychic process of struggle against the disease or of ongoing resilience induced by the experience of a serious illness? The usual interview procedure was therefore relaxed to respect the probable loophole created by the telephone exchange. This allowed interviewees to address unforeseen themes and allowed the stories to be unusually dispersed. The difficulty was to avoid falling into a posture that could be perceived as psychological support that would have engaged us. The transparency of our posture as a researcher and not as a caregiver and the vigilance on the feelings expressed seemed to us to guarantee the ethical nature of our approach: if the psychological process triggered by the interview indicated a need for support that we could not have identified, we considered referring the person to competent professionals. This situation did not arise.

Is there a professional limit of scientific research to empathy? Empathy is an ability to understand how others feel and to signify to them in the current relationship. Since the investigator in this field is a former caregiver, the challenge was to find out how the data collection was limited to ICS research without switching to the confidences obtained through caregiving skills. It is part of the imposed reflexivity that preserved an ethical tension during the work. Interested in the constitution of stratagems set up by Internet users to federate solidarity or to develop expertise, we focused on the circuits developed beyond the forums by Internet users. To what extent then should the public/private boundary not be breached?

5.3.3. *Protecting respondents*

For the field related to therapeutic cannabis, which was illegal in France at the time this research was conducted, and which was regulated differently in some states of the United States and Canada, the approach of the user–patient communities was a definite difficulty for the researcher. Legislation prohibiting the use of cannabis in France since the 1970s forbids its use in a positive light[6]. In the end, it is forbidden to talk about it, because talking about a drug implies talking about the motivations for consumption, such as the search for a better well-being that would erase the risk/benefit ratio concerning addiction and dependence. Beyond a dimension qualified as "recreational", cannabis is officially recognized as useful in cancer treatment. For example, it is used for the indication "Supportive care in oncology" by the Comité Scientifique Specialisé Temporaire, CSST (French Temporary Specialized Scientific Committee) of the Agence Nationale de la Sureté du Médicament (French National Agency for the Safety of Medicines)[7]. The favorable opinion issued by the CSST on the experimentation of therapeutic cannabis in France was based on studies concerning its use in anti-cancer treatments, making it possible to reduce the side effects associated with chemotherapy. It is in this paradoxical info-communication context, where the expert voice, muzzled by legislation, seems inaudible in the face of the deployment of an experiential counter-discourse extolling the therapeutic benefits of cannabis that ethical questions about the protection of respondents appear particularly heuristic.

We did not attempt to meet with stakeholders from the forums in which they spoke. The clandestine nature of their practice has made them

6 Article L3421-4 of the French Public Health Code states: "Provocation to commit the offence provided for in Article L. 3421-1 or one of the offences provided for in Articles 222-34 to 222-39 of the Criminal Code, even if such provocation has not been followed up, or the fact of presenting these offences in a favorable light, shall be punishable by five years' imprisonment and a fine of 75,000 euros".

7 Comité Scientifique Spécialisé Temporaire "évaluation de la pertinence et de la faisabilité de la mise à disposition du cannabis thérapeutique en France". Therapeutic Cannabis: Experimental Project. June 19, 2019 version.

suspicious of any type of meeting emanating from the forums in which they participate. It should be noted that police operations have already targeted these communities[8] and that they protect themselves from any intervention by the offline world in their online exchanges. "For your security, be careful not to divulge information that could compromise your anonymity (geographical location, known pseudonym, etc.)", as stated in the Cannaweed.com forum rules. Disclosure of their identity not only involves a violation of their privacy, but also puts them at risk of judicial condemnation. The anonymity of the members of these forums is cultivated to a regular profile change for some contributors.

Although participants use pseudonyms, we made the choice to conceal them in the pre-exploitation data collection and analysis of exchanges using false pseudonyms in order to protect the interviewee's digital identity. A symbolic capital can be attached to this identity, which ensures the latter's status as an online expert that should not be devalued. Also, we avoided including verbatim quotes that would have made the participants easily recognizable. A "fabrication" citation was thus put into practice by combining and reorganizing elements [MAR 12] so that participants could not be identified. Indeed, our corpus being partly accessible to the public online, a search based on the original verbatim would make it possible to find certain messages and participants, thus breaking anonymity.

5.3.4. *Protecting researchers in controversies and emotionally engaging research*

Interviewing people with cancer requires two forms of protection: the first, that of the participants, concerns medical and personal data and their vulnerability. Indeed, with a few clues, it can be easy to find people online. The second concerns the researchers themselves. Indeed, researchers often think about protecting their participants, but forget to protect themselves by applying basic privacy principles. We have avoided publicly posting announcements on the forums, preferring to contact participants ourselves after reading their messages and profiles.

Online public speaking, if anything, as a form of interaction ritual aimed at seeking the approval of the rest of the community for its integration and

8 http://www.leparisien.fr/faits-divers/coup-de-filet-parmi-les-cultivateurs-de-cannabis-a-domicile-06-05-2011-1438177.php.

thus access to the voice of the interviewees, subjects the researcher to the risk of controversy. This is particularly true for socially acute health issues, such as therapeutic cannabis. In a tense social climate, in which digital social networks are becoming counter-models of the normative ideal of the virtual community, built upon the ethics of discussion [HAB 85], generosity and recognition [GAL 14], the researcher must polarize the information content he or she is supposed to observe, by tracing its origin and understanding its production context.

Moreover, with regard to the necessary protection of the researcher, the contents of health forums can quickly prove to be morbid and anxiety-provoking. Good emotion management will then be necessary to avoid being overwhelmed by too much negativity. But an ICS researcher does not *a priori* have the expertise neither to receive the suffering of others nor to manage all the emotions induced by this context. The collective dimension of ICS research in the field of care and health may therefore be conducive to the necessary distance. Sharing the evolution of the different investigations makes it easier and allows us to put into perspective not the suffering of others, but the possible emotionality resulting from the stories heard. This is the choice we made by organizing formal and informal exchanges between project team members to "put at distance" the risks of harmful emotional involvement. Empirical and methodological ethics therefore imply communicative caution and reflective collegiality.

5.4. Conclusion

In this proposal, we wanted to propose a reflexive look at the researcher's field action in online socialization spaces. We have chosen, beyond the classical propositions on methodologies and their dedicated epistemological context, to question these practices from an ethical point of view. How should researchers summon principles, respect and humility with regard to the perimeters of their observations and the use made of their field data? From this perspective, we restricted the scope of our ethical questioning to what we have called "empirical and methodological ethics".

As a result, we have not embraced the whole of scientific ethics in the field of health and, in general, in HSS. We have not, for example, systematically studied the legal institutionalization of empirical and methodological ethics in different cultural contexts, particularly in

French-speaking Canada, which is an important field of observation for our objects. Similarly, we have not questioned the role of social demand, which is the driving force behind much of the research in this field, whether this social demand comes from private companies, local authorities or State agencies such as the Regional Health Agencies in France. The ethical questions then asked of the researcher thus begin by questioning who is he/she working for? What are the risks of instrumentalizing the results it produces? Although we have been able to address the question of the use of data collected during empirical approaches and the protection of respondents (even in the standards for storing the data collected, as is already the case in the conditions for validating empirical protocols imposed by the University of Geneva in Switzerland[9]), the fact remains that the generalization of contract research, in project mode, requires researchers to maintain a reflective distance that cannot be satisfied with a purely epistemological stance.

From then on, the critical and reflexive dimension, a real ethical "safeguard", is imposed on the researcher in the sense that it questions the strategies of organized and/or institutionalized actors who either benefit from the social practices observed or who try to rationalize for the sake of effectiveness or efficiency. By directly integrating this socio-economic and political contextualization in the very construction of the research object, we articulate the micro-dimension of the observations of info-communication practices of patients or caregivers (or even health professionals) to the meso standardization resulting from organizational managerial standards or community management policies, positioning the whole in strategic state or economic macro-stakes. Thus, in the era of big data, the collective awareness of the societal issues of data governance cannot be foreign to the professional activity of the researcher. The use of "patient" data for commercial purposes or health system optimization is something that ICS research in the health field, from our perspective, cannot ignore.

In healthcare, work conducted in ICS can question the computerization of healthcare institutions, the new digital mediations of knowledge and the tensions concerning the emerging amateur or lay forms of expertise that they entail, or online social support or injunctions to "empower" the patient (to be an actor in his/her health) in a restricted public space at the heart of health

9 https://www.unige.ch/fti/files/9515/4503/4057/Gestion__donnees_de_recherche_Commission__ethique_FTI.pdf.

democracy. All these subjects call for reflective and critical caution which, based on the empirical and methodological scientific ethics we have outlined here, must help us to propose a responsible production of knowledge.

5.5. References

[BAL 93] BALAZS G., BOURDIEU P., "L'interrogatoire", in BOURDIEU P. (ed.), *La Misère du monde*, Le Seuil, Paris, 1993.

[BAR 13] BARATS C., *Manuel d'analyse du web en Sciences Humaines et Sociales*, 2nd edition, Armand Colin, Paris, 2013.

[BOU 91] BOURDONCLE R., "La professionnalisation des enseignants: analyses sociologiques anglaises et américaines", *Revue française de pédagogie*, no. 94, pp. 73–92, 1991.

[CAR 04] CARATINI S., *Les non-dits de l'anthropologie*, Presses Universitaires de France, Paris, 2004.

[COU 14] COULON A., *L'ethnométhodologie*, Presses Universitaires de France, Paris, 2014.

[FOU 16] FOURNIER C., WINANCE M., "Questionnements éthiques dans les recherches qualitatives en santé", in KIVITS J., BALARD F., FOURNIER C. *et al.* (eds), *Les recherches qualitatives en santé*, Armand Colin, Paris, 2016.

[GAL 14] GALIBERT O., "Approche communicationnelle et organisationnelle des enjeux du Community Management", *Communication et Organisation*, no. 46, pp. 265–278, 2014.

[GAR 07] GARFINKEL H., *Recherches en ethnométhodologie [1967]*, Presses Universitaires de France, Paris, 2007.

[HIN 05] HINE C., *Virtual Methods: Issues in Social Research on the Internet*, Berg Publishers, Oxford, 2005.

[HUM 17] HUMPHREYS L., *Tearoom Trade: Impersonal Sex in Public Places*, Routledge, New York, 2017.

[LAH 92] LAHIRE B., "Précisions sur la manière sociologique de traiter du "sens": quelques remarques concernant l'ethnométhodologie", *Langage & société*, vol. 59, no. 1, pp. 73–89, 1992.

[LAT 13] LATZKO-TOTH G., PROULX S., "Enjeux éthiques de la recherche sur le Web", in BARATS C. (ed.), *Manuel d'analyse du web en Sciences Humaines et Sociales*, Armand Colin, Paris, 2013.

[MAR 12] MARKHAM A., "Fabrication as ethical practice: Qualitative inquiry in ambiguous internet contexts", *Information, Communication & Society*, no. 3, pp. 334–353, 2012.

[MIL 63] MILGRAM S., "Behavioral study of obedience", *Journal of Abnormal and Social Psychology*, no. 67, pp. 371–378, 1963.

[RIC 04] RICOEUR P., "Ethique", in CANTO-SPERBER M. (ed.), *Dictionnaire d'éthique et de philosophie morale*, Presses Universitaires de France, Paris, 2004.

[SIR 04] SIROUX D., "Déontologie", in CANTO-SPERBER M. (ed.), *Dictionnaire d'éthique et de philosophie morale*, Presses Universitaires de France, Paris, 2004.

[THO 12] THOËR C., MILLERAND F., MYLES D. *et al.*, "Enjeux éthiques de la recherche sur les forums Internet portant sur l'utilisation des médicaments à des fins non médicales", *Communiquer - Revue de communication sociale et publique*, no. 7, pp. 1–22, 2012.

[VAS 08] VASSY C., KELLER R., "Faut-il contrôler les aspects éthiques de la recherche en sciences sociales, et comment ?", *Mouvements*, nos 55–56, pp. 128–141, 2008.

[WIL 88] WILKINSON S., "The role of reflexivity in feminist psychology", *Women's Studies International Forum*, vol. 11, pp. 493–502, 1988.

6

Action Research at La Poste to Prevent the Psychosocial Risks Associated with Digital Acculturation

6.1. Introduction

As a social worker at the Toulouse financial center of the La Poste Group, we conducted between 2013 and 2016 action research (AR) as part of a PhD in information and communication sciences (ICSs). The purpose of this study was to consider the prevention of psychosocial risks related to digital acculturation. Social workers play a special role in developing the quality of life and occupational health of postal workers. They occupy a privileged position to address issues related to change management and the prevention of psychosocial risks, in a context of generalized crisis and the evolution of strategic communication plans. AR is here adapted to the work context, since it presupposes the real space of an organization and the symbolic space of a project of renewal:

> "The framework is that of human activities or work engaged in an indefinite future. The aim remains the expected transformation, the expected change, the crisis to be induced or calmed, the future values to be promoted" [BER 95, p. 13].

Thus, our research questioned the professional practices of an organization in a context of digital change and ultimately aimed to improve working conditions. The study of the prevention of psychosocial risks

---

Chapter written by Emilie BLANC.

through the prism of communication appears all the more relevant since, following two suicides by executives in the workplace, Jean-Paul Bailly, then Chairman and CEO of La Poste Group, launched a "Great Dialogue" on life and well-being at work in March 2012. The aim was to open up avenues for reflection and action enabling the company to become a pioneer in improving well-being at work in a context of permanent change. It therefore seemed interesting to us to select the "Great Dialogue" as an object of study, in order to analyze in greater depth the communication strategies at work.

To do so, we decided to register in one of the fields of ICS, namely that of organizational communication. The communication "of" and "in" organizations is the subject of numerous empirical works [BOU 08b] and therefore seems relevant to analyze an innovative device such as the "Great Dialogue". Among the six approaches distinguished within this field [GRO 11], we retained the so-called "constitutive" approach, which considers that organizations are continually (re)building themselves. What was undertaken was then dependent on relationships that (re)configured and (re)arranged organizations. There was not a constitution but constitutions of the organization. The project of our AR was therefore to give employees a voice on digital transformation issues so that they could become co-constructors of communication and organization, with communication becoming "organizational".

In this chapter, we wish to conduct reflexive feedback on AR and the method used. In order to do this, we will first go back over some of the characteristics of AR. We then present our various data collection techniques. Finally, we conclude with some ethical questions about the work carried out.

6.2. The relevance of action research to prevent psychosocial risks

It was the psychosociologist Kurt Lewin [LÉW 46] who between 1940 and 1945 formalized AR. It is, according to him, an implied research aimed at transforming social practices and it is through the co-construction of meaning, which results from confrontation and dialogue, that reflection on practice is possible. AR is a process that takes place in collaboration between researchers, organizational actors and sometimes users in order to produce scientific knowledge about the situations under study. It differs from basic research because it involved research that is conducted in the field for operational purposes. The aim being therapeutic, it intervenes on social practices in order to transform them. It tries to change social reality. The framework of intervention is that of a work engaged in a future which is not defined at the beginning. In any case, action always presupposes the real space of an organization, the involvement of its members and the symbolic space of a renewal project.

Although there are many variants of AR, several common points can be noted:

> "AR is a process; it is a research approach aimed at solving concrete problems in real-life situations; it is implemented through collaboration between researchers and company players [...]; its objective is to produce scientific knowledge on the situations studied" [JOU 09, p. 5].

The starting point of the research process is to identify and define a concrete problem: this is the diagnostic phase. Then you have to plan, i.e. consider different forms of action, to solve the problem. Once the action has been carried out, it must be evaluated and the overall results identified. This process is cyclical. In other words, the stages of the cycle are run through several times and learning is done in a progressive manner. The actors of the company are in the middle of this iterative process, since they effectively participate in the action "while taking into consideration the organization of which they are only representatives" [JOU 09, p. 5].

The principle of AR is applicable to a variety of settings, including organizational settings. Today, the human and social sciences are regularly called upon in professional circles to produce knowledge by shedding light, for example, on the conduct and practices of actors. And, given practitioners' expectations of a discourse that guarantees the act and of knowledge that can be immediately operationalized, AR remains more relevant than ever:

> "Associating the actor's research with that of the academic is rich in interest, because it means accepting the contradictory debate, the dialectic necessary for distancing, it means conjugating the logic of proximity of the actor with the capacity of critical distance of the researcher" [BOU 08a, p. 30].

In this context, due to the nature of their research projects, ICS can be used to address a wide range of issues relating to change management, crisis management, quality approaches, risk prevention, strategic communication plans, etc.

A study of AR conducted in the field of communication of organizations in ICS [BOU 08b] reveals a wide variety of theoretical borrowings and methodological experiences. Implementation does not depend solely on rational criteria defined *a priori*, but is, on the contrary, strongly adjusted to the specificities of the field and the expectations of the actors concerned. Thus, from the outset, the application for AR can take different forms, depending on whether it comes from a field project or a research contract. Then, the object can be progressively delimited with a constrained choice of methods and difficult access to information. The statuses and roles of the actors involved may also interfere. In the course of his or her commitment and fieldwork, the researcher may be confronted with misunderstandings, individual and collective resistance, and local contingencies... Finally, the concrete course of the different phases of an AR, up to the restitution of results, may evolve according to its effects on the organization and the actors.

Given these points of tension, it is easier to understand why it is relatively rare to be able to apply a pre-established approach, such as a "recipe". Because the method needs to be adjusted on a case-by-case basis, AR involves, perhaps even more than other approaches, an inevitable "tinkering" [LÉV 62]. It is, moreover, these "arrangements" that would make it possible to get to the heart of the field and ultimately produce knowledge for both the scientific community and practitioners, without betraying the latter. However, while it is essential to take into account the difficulties in order to adapt to the constraints, this does not mean reducing the relevance and scientificity of the research. In fact, a global and therefore complex methodological reflection is essential both in the choice of techniques and in their implementation.

However, it is rare to find in-depth analyses and/or specific examples in the literature of the practical conditions of methodological deployment in the field during AR. Similarly, the detailed presentation of the difficulties encountered and the analysis of the consequences on the results remain mostly fragmented. Under an agreed formalism, the iterative aspect of the investigative process, with its trial and error and "tinkering", is generally overlooked, although it inevitably constitutes the daily routine of all involved and applied research. This is why we propose in the following section to present the method finally implemented for our AR.

6.3. What method in action research prevents psychosocial risks?

In order to support the management of change and thus act on the prevention of psychosocial risks related to digital acculturation, we postulated that our AR needed to initiate a collective reflection by and for employees. However, when the researcher transforms research into an act of collective production and knowledge, he/she goes through phases of deconstruction and reconstruction. We therefore sought to collect and produce different types of information: on the digital practices of social workers, on the challenges in their daily professional activity and on possible optimization processes at work; on support for the "digital acculturation" of the most disadvantaged employees and those retiring; on optimizing the use of digital technology for employees who are far away from the Center and who are returning home, particularly due to illness. In order to do so, we articulated several types of collection and analysis according to their relevance: documentary, quantitative and qualitative.

Documentary collection is an essential step, where possible, even before the field research. The ethnologist Marcel Maget (1909–1994) considered: "Except in cases of extreme urgency, the investigation is never undertaken without a review of the available documentation on the chosen subject" [COM 07, p. 12]. As far as we were concerned, we collected minutes of meetings, internal journals, extracts from the intranet of the Financial Center and La Poste Group, and historical works on La Poste.

Then, a quantitative method – through the administration of a questionnaire and statistical analysis – was used three times: twice by the "practitioners–learners–researchers" in social work [MAC 01] in order to collect data on the personal and professional digital practices of social workers in all financial services; once by the communication department, in order to evaluate the digital practices of the employees of the Toulouse Financial Center. The questionnaires were distributed in digital format, either by email or via the Center's intranet. These questionnaires, used for exploratory purposes, made it possible in particular to obtain information on the different profiles of social workers in order to reflect on the implementation of actions.

Finally, a qualitative approach was used to study the optimization of the use of digital technology for employees who were away from the Center and who had returned home, notably due to illness. Initially, semi-directive interviewing was used because it encouraged "confident expression" [COM 07, p. 25], as spontaneous as possible, particularly through reminders. While the maintenance guide specified pre-established themes, it enabled the introduction of its own dynamics. Moreover, the interview seemed particularly suitable for gathering the testimony of collaborators with a particular experience. In total, more than 20 semi-structured interviews were conducted in three different financial centers. In a second phase, these interviews were supplemented by a group interview at the Toulouse financial center, in the form of a discussion forum, so that these employees could exchange and share their experiences. The theoretical challenge was to collect a collective word, produced by the interaction. This type of interview was a valuable technique to allow the expression of particularly stigmatized or inferior groups, such as, for example, employees returning due to illness. Most often, the group pre-existed as such before the interview. Within the framework of our AR, it was of an experimental type and brought together on a basis other than inter-knowledge for the circumstance. However, there needed to be sufficient social homogeneity, for example, a common experience, for the discussion to be productive. The professional group in our AR was made up of employees from the Toulouse Financial Center, who had the same experience of remote and returning employees.

Other techniques were initially considered. We felt, for example, that the collection of "life stories" from employees would have provided insight into the experiences of the various organizational changes. However, the human resources department did not want us to do this so as not to "stir up" a past that was still painful for some. This type of methodological compromise ultimately raises ethical questions about the position of the researcher engaged in AR.

6.4. Action research for ethical questions

For Paul Ricoeur, ethics can be considered as "the objective of a good life with and for others in just institutions" [RIC 96, p. 202].

> "Here we find the thorny question of measuring what is right and what is true, which invites us to reflect epistemologically as well as to evaluate without complacency our activities in the production of organizational knowledge" [BOU 08b p. 14].

In the context of organizational intervention, ethics concerns both the analysis of situations and the recursive loop with actors modifying visions and potentially actions [RIC 08]. Ethics therefore obliges the researcher to take responsibility for his or her choices of research and action, as well as to evaluate the consequences of the results before explaining and justifying them. Reflecting on ethics is therefore thinking about the very heart of the researcher's job, their responsibility and freedom, their values and aims, their positions.

Like any researcher working in a company, we were confronted with ethical questions, whether it was on the issues of AR, on the method, on the researcher's position or on his/her relationship with the field. These issues became even more acute in an evolving organizational context where actors developed opportunistic strategies according to their interests. In order to address some of the ethical issues during AR, we distinguished three stages: upstream with the negotiation of research objectives, during the conduct of the research, and downstream with the presentation of results and the evaluation of the actions carried out.

Among the tensions that may exist during the AR preparation phase, the researcher must identify, evacuate or rework some of the presuppositions that pre-determine the categories to be studied. In order to allow the co-construction of a problem to be processed, it is necessary to cross the perspectives and projects of researchers, sponsors and even actors. The dialogue makes it possible to frame the situation, to confront professional realities, to find a balance between the issues of "truth" [JAS 61] and operationality, and to define an intervention plan. Conflicts of interpretation as well as paradoxical injunctions are therefore not uncommon. The assessment of the situation thus leads to a mediation of the values, experiences and symbolic forms involved. However, the agreements found should not be considered as stable structures since they can be modified during the investigation.

In AR, the evolution of organizational arrangements requires a constant cross-fertilization of expert and lay knowledge, a construction–deconstruction–

reconstruction of the processes at work, and the consideration of the changing positions of the stakeholders (researchers, sponsors and actors in the organization). The articulation between “actor–researcher” and “action–research” can then become complex. For Benoît Cordelier, “becoming a member, in the sense of Harold Garfinkel, remains a source of tension in which the strategic and operational logics of the departments largely condition the operating methods and analyses” [BOU 08b p. 11]. The researcher’s commitment is therefore likely to be tested both by his or her status as a stakeholder in the situation and by the play of alliances that can make the terrain unstable. Being ourselves integrated as a social worker in this environment, we did not have to justify our presence to the actors concerned. Our place and our role therefore represented an opportunity and an interesting occasion to launch such an approach. But then, it was a question of accepting to “juggle” between academic and field requirements.

Downstream, AR – as we have already explained – is part of an evolution of representations and induces actions that modify the organization.

> “In synergy with their environment and the history that inhabits them, participatory action research (PAR) practitioners, armed with their knowledge but also with their ability to support, guide social change in such a way as to enable social actors to better adapt to the complex issues and challenges that challenge them” [CHE 13 p. 3].

The restitution of results first to the sponsor and then to the actors is therefore likely to become a feedback game influenced by the culture of the organization and in particular by its social norms of acceptability. It may also give rise to negotiations between the obligation of confidentiality and the public disclosure of results. Finally, following the presentation of the results of PLAR, unexpected effects may occur such as, for example, the dissolution of collectives or discouragement.

6.5. Conclusion

During this AR, which was the core of our thesis in ICS, we found, contrary to what we had initially assumed, that digital acculturation did not represent a psychosocial risk factor for employees. This situation is, among other things, due, in our opinion, to an adapted support from the communication department. The actions undertaken, such as the organization of "digital breakfasts", have played a protective role against psychosocial risks. In addition, social workers, realizing that some employees might have difficulties in their use of technology, have created "digital workshops" to support them. They were primary prevention actions for psychosocial risks. Finally, we found that social workers' digital technology practices may contribute to their own protection from psychosocial risks. For example, their regular email exchanges allow them to help each other and break some form of isolation.

However, different limits are emerging. We choose to develop only two. First of all, these results arise from a particular context, as is all research in the human and social sciences. Our results are only valid in a given context and the results would probably be different today. For example, the social workers developed the use of digital technologies also because their technical coordinator was absent for several months. Today, however, this professional has returned and the social workers have changed due to retirements. The group dynamics and uses of digital would therefore be different. The second limitation concerns our status. As a social worker, we were indeed constrained by company policy and by the ethical obligations specific to our profession. For example, the collaborators interviewed on their return to the Center after being away for several months due to illness, among other reasons, were interviewed not only by the researcher but also, at the same time, by "their" social worker. This may have had an effect on their attitudes and responses. Secondly, when analyzing the results, we did not adopt a radical critical perspective on either the prevention of psychosocial risks or the participatory aspect of the "Great Dialogue".

6.6. References

[BER 95] BERTHON J.-F., *La Recherche-Action*, PUF, Paris, 1995.

[BLA 16] BLANC E., Du "Grand Dialogue" au quotidien numérique: des stratégies de communication à La Poste, PhD thesis, Université Nice Sophia Antipolis, Université Côte d'Azur, 2016.

[BOU 08a] BOUQUET B., GARCETTE C., *Assistante sociale aujourd'hui*, Maloine, Paris, 2008.

[BOU 08b] BOUZON A., MEYER V., *La communication des organisations, entre recherche et action*, L'Harmattan, Paris, 2008.

[CHE 13] CHEVALIER J., BUCKLES D., BOURASSA M., *Guide de la recherche-action, la planification et l'évaluation participatives*, SAS Dialogue, Ottawa, 2013.

[COM 07] COMBESSIE J.-C., *La méthode en sociologie*, La Découverte, Paris, 2007.

[COR 08] CORDELIER B., MARIE-MONTAGNAC H., "Conduire le changement organisationnel?", *Communication & Organisation*, no. 33, pp. 8–16, 2008.

[DEC 07] DE CEGLIE A., Du réseau à la communauté d'apprenants. Quelle dynamique du lien social pour faire œuvre?, PhD thesis, Université Aix-Marseille 1, 2007.

[DUB 87] DUBOST J., *L'intervention psychosociologique*, PUF, Paris, 1987.

[GRO 11] GROSJEAN S., BONNEVILLE L., *La communication organisationnelle. Approches, processus et enjeu*, Chenelière Education, Quebec, 2011.

[JAS 82] JASPERS K., *Introduction à la philosophie*, Editions Plon, Paris, 1982.

[JOU 09] JOUISON-LAFFITTE E., "La recherche-action: oubliée de la recherche dans le domaine de l'entreprenariat", *Revue de l'entrepreneuriat*, vol. 8, no. 1, pp. 1–35, 2009.

[LAB 10] LABERGE Y., "Interactionnisme symbolique, ethnométhodologie et microsociologie", *Recherches sociologiques et anthropologiques*, no. 40-2, pp. 151–156, 2010.

[LAP 91] LAPASSADE G., *L'ethno-sociologie. Analyse institutionnelle*, Meridiens Klincksieck, Paris, 1991.

[LÉV 62] LÉVI-STRAUSS C., *La Pensée sauvage*, Éditions Plon, Paris, 1962.

[LÉW 46] LÉWIN K., "Action research and minority problems", *Journal of Social Issues*, vol. 2, no. 4, pp. 34–46, 1946.

[MAC 01] MACKIEWICZ M.-P., *Praticien et chercheur, Parcours dans le champ social*, L'Harmattan, Paris, 2001.

[RIC 08] RICHARD V., "Des questionnements convergents sur l'éthique", in BOUZON A., MEYER V. (eds), *La communication des organisations, entre recherche et action*, L'Harmattan, Paris, pp. 227–231, 2008.

[RIC 96] RICOEUR P., *Soi-même comme un autre*, Le Seuil, Paris, 1996.

[VAC 08] VACHER B., "La communication organisationnelle en France: en formalisme et débrouillardise: Une histoire de paradoxe à décrypter", in ROGOJINARU A., BOUZON A. (eds), *Fondements de la communication des organisations: tendances internationales*, Tritonic, Bucharest, pp. 33–56, 2008.

PART 3

Thinking Approaches to Health Research in a Digital Context

7

Interests and Limitations of Interdisciplinary Research in a Living Lab to Meet the Needs of Senior Citizens

7.1. Introduction

For several years, French public policies have focused on the implementation of home support systems adapted to the elderly. Depending on the actors concerned – the scientific community and the medical profession, private companies, associations – the acceptability and the stakes of aging differ.

Old age can thus be thought of as the result of scientific progress in the field of health, a market within the Silver economy, a context favorable to the prescriptions of "aging well", which aims to prevent, support and offer older people "the steps on the road to successful aging" [AQU 08, p. 45]. The focus on age, in order to define solutions for the support and care of senior citizens, often leads to a standardized offer through centralized planning [MEM 08]. Thus, the needs of the elderly are considered in relation to the dependency, loss of autonomy and "burden" that they would represent for society. The discourse on the "inevitable lapse" of old age can make us forget its social definition [MAR 00]. According to a social definition, age is not sufficient to qualify the ways of aging, given the diversity of ways of arranging the home, using outside services, maintaining social relations, carrying out activities, etc. Thus, it is not enough to qualify the ways of aging, in view of the diversity of ways of arranging the home, using outside

---

Chapter written by Elizabeth BOUGEOIS and Hélène GERMAIN.

services, maintaining social relations, carrying out activities, etc. [MEM 13]. Seen in this way, aging can become a "project" and not a destiny [LAL 91]. This cleavage between social definitions, on the one hand, and economic and medical definitions, on the other hand, echoes "the reflection of a paradoxical society torn between individualism and solidarity" [ENN 13, p. 34], where the notion of "independence" is prescribed by institutions "to the detriment of the recognition of dependence in its original meaning as a mode of relationship between individuals, interdependence and the foundation of social cohesion" [ENN 13, p. 31].

Current public research funding policies encourage researchers to focus on technologies to bypass the loss of autonomy: these are considered likely to enhance the independence and well-being of older people [VIG 17]. Technical and home automation devices have been emerging since the 1980s. In particular, they developed during the 2000s with the introduction of remote assistance for the elderly – mainly symbolized by the necklace to call in the event of a fall – remote management, which promotes the transmission of information and/or the management of remote services and the installation of remote alarms to ensure the safety of property [BON 08]. Technological innovation today mainly concerns artificial intelligence and the Internet of Things.

However, these technologies, largely developed according to a medicalized view of old age, are criticized for not meeting the needs of the people concerned and therefore not always being accepted by them. Thus, disability compensation is often thought out according to the gestures, uses and representations of able-bodied people, which leads to the design of "validocentered" devices [GAR 12, MAY 17]. Also, the use of technological tools can generate fears, as expressed by the elderly: fear of stigmatization, fear of being considered even more of a burden to society, fear of loss of autonomy precisely because of the palliation provided by a system, which can replace the user's activity, fear of loss of sociability [POR 13].

The appropriation or non-utilization of a technology thus depends partly on identity, relational and psychological factors specific to each individual [CLE 16]. The consideration of older people as a passive population in the face of new technologies is unfounded: on the contrary, they prove to be actors of change [MEM 08], by showing inventiveness and adaptation to daily life. Let's go beyond the postulate that older people resist novelty [CAR 99]: the difficulties of use encountered generally depend on "product-specific ergonomic deficiencies" and not on incapacities often attributed to users [BOU 02].

So how can the relevance of the technologies developed be assessed? What scientific methods should be used to meet the needs of older people? In this context, collaborative action research can be an interesting tool, in that it allows the participation, in the study presented in this chapter, of those concerned by the proposal and implementation of adapted technical solutions. The action research approach would also promote "democratic governance of science and technology" [BON 13]. The purpose of collaborative action research is to overcome "a contradiction between the way research is conducted, the dominant paradigms and the interests and needs of populations ... and of the researchers themselves" [LEC 13, p. 73]. The particularity of this research is to develop participatory scientific methods "that seek and need to be tested and evaluated" [LES 15]. Through these practices is established "a learning process for both the researcher and the actor, a process in which theory and practice, thought and action are not distinct, but associated" [WCC 01, p. 21]. Thus, the design of technological tools, in this type of participatory research, tends to move away from the technology push models, which consist of putting products on the market without having verified their concrete usefulness or including the people concerned in the creation process [FRA 10].

In this perspective, Living Labs in Health and Autonomy (LLSA, from the French *Living Labs en Santé et Autonomie*) are developing as innovative organizations whose objective is to co-design, with users, technical solutions for personal assistance, based on citizen participation and open innovation [BER 17]. This user-centered participatory design method aims to redefine the roles of actors in "public–private–people-partnerships", in which the people surveyed are considered as experts in a field that directly concerns them. The designation of the expert-user role can be controversial and its legitimacy is not always well accepted in power–knowledge relationships [TER 17]. However, the position of user-expert is fully legitimized by the knowledge of use, i.e. "the knowledge that an individual or a group has of their immediate and daily environment, based on experience and proximity" [NEZ 13]. Here, the expert is a specialist in "his/her particular case", not in old age and health in general, but in what their set experience [GOF 64], allows them to express, in a contextualized manner, about aging and health [PAG 14].

The solicitation of user-experts in LLSAs makes it possible to gather the needs and knowledge of senior citizens in a context that promotes trust with researchers through the recognition of reciprocal skills. This status allows respondents to share their "critical reflections" [STO 12] on research and technical devices developed *in vitro*. This reconsideration of experimentation by the people surveyed allows researchers to improve their scientific practice and the design of technical devices [STO 12]. The success of this participatory research is based, therefore, on the involvement and commitment of the various stakeholders.

On the basis of two successive studies carried out in LLSAs, we will see how the processes of interest and involvement of three types of actors (user-experts, researchers from different disciplines) were formed, as well as the development of their reflections on the method and technologies developed in LLSAs. The first study concerns senior citizens experiencing, in an LLSA, the use of a technical device to palliate the loss of autonomy. The second aims to reconsider the multimodal observation method developed for the first. After presenting these two studies, we explain the three forms of reconsideration implemented by the respondents, the researchers and a sociology trainee.

7.2. Reconsidering a Living Lab study: the centrality of user-experts

The two studies on which this chapter is based are unique, in that they were conducted in an LLSA by a multidisciplinary team of six researchers and one trainee in Information and Communication Sciences and Technologies (ICST), three women researchers and one trainee in Human and Social Sciences (HSS), and a geriatrician. ICST researchers specialize in sensor engineering, networks and human–machine interaction. They are behind the creation of the LLSA. In the first study, they called upon researchers in HSS (sociology, anthropology and information and communication sciences) to define and implement a multimodal, quantitative and qualitative observation method in a controlled environment. The geriatrician joined the team during the second study. We can already note the gendered dimension of scientific disciplines and the minority in number of HSS.

7.2.1. *Senior citizens and new technologies in a controlled environment*

The first study aimed at collecting and analyzing the uses and needs of senior citizens in new technologies, via two questionnaires, the execution of a scenario of taking over a domotized universe in LLSA and a 10-minute semi-directive interview. The only criterion for the inclusion of respondents was that they were over 60 years of age. A total of 146 people participated. A first questionnaire made it possible to identify the socio-professional category of the participants, their current and past family and social living conditions, their health constraints, their knowledge and use of connected technological objects.

Participants then visited a home that was domotized and connected. They were presented with the different equipment (bedroom–toilet light path; height-adjustable furniture, etc.) and the control methods (switches, touch table, voice control) of this equipment. The participants, individually supervised, tested this equipment using the three proposed ways of ordering. They would then, alone, perform a scenario for about 10 minutes (getting up and the actions that usually follow it in their daily lives). They were, at that time, filmed and observed, their words were recorded, as well as the actions carried out, the ways of ordering these actions and the actimetric data. This was followed by a short interview to gather their views and to question any changes in their perceptions or representations of digital technologies, using a short questionnaire to qualify and quantify any such changes.

During the experiments, different degrees of ease in the use of technological tools were observed by the researchers. Some participants showed confidence with the proposed technical devices, using all the interaction modalities and technical functions of the LLSA – even simulating a fall to meet the assumed expectations of researchers and to verify the potentialities of the controlled environment. Other participants felt uncomfortable and did not dare to use certain technical devices because of their unfamiliarity, or commented on their actions as they were performed. For these people, this experimentation sometimes proved to be “an exercise where we were told to come and go”, revealing a feeling of “looking silly” in this new environment. Some felt they had played an acting role during these experiments with an imposed scenario, sometimes feeling “under the influence of instructions” or embarrassed by the fact that they knew they were being observed. Also, feelings of discomfort were expressed, due to an environment, the LLSA, deemed “too medicalized”. Participation in the experiment sometimes forced the people surveyed to immerse themselves in an anticipation that was disturbing for them: “the most difficult thing was to imagine myself as an invalid, who could no longer come and go as he pleased … this was very complicated”.

These findings were analyzed by the research team as specific elements for defining observation limits in LLSA. As the controlled environment constitutes a passage, an intermediate step towards the ecological environment of people, i.e. their home, it proved necessary to reconsider the mixed qualitative–quantitative methodological device implemented, to question in depth the senior participants and to study more closely the stakes of scientific interdisciplinarity.

7.2.2. *The second study or how to reconsider research practices*

In order to meet these different objectives, it was decided to reconsider the first study through the prism of the methodological framework and what underlies it. This reconsideration was carried out by three types of actors (users-experts, researchers, student trainee in master’s degree in sociology) and was done in two stages: a focus group observed by the members of the research team, with six volunteers (one man and five women) who participated in the first study, then a semi-directive interview with each of them, in their own homes. The commitment of the people surveyed is formalized by a verbal and moral contract with the research team.

The researchers’ reflexive feedback on their method of observation was carried out through a risk analysis, a methodological tool proposed by the team’s geriatrician. This tool is based on the assumption that there are methodological risks in conducting a scientific study [BON 13]. The objective here was to familiarize the entire team with this tool in order to build, in a second step, specifications presenting the identified risks and corrective measures, in order to envisage the deployment of the observation method in the homes of the participants.

The trainee recruited as part of her second year of her master’s degree in sociology observed the team of researchers during all their work meetings and questioned each of them in order to learn about their representations of old age, the elderly, dependency, the home and new technologies. Her work also consisted in observing the interactions between scientists and senior participants and between researchers from different disciplinary backgrounds, in order to obtain an organizational diagnosis. More specifically, her work has made it possible to identify, in the discourse of the people surveyed and the researchers, convergences and divergences in representations relating to the phenomena studied. Putting them into perspective made it possible to clarify certain postures.

Researchers and senior citizens surveyed thus share a curiosity about object design, said to be smart. On the user-expert side, a lot of hope is placed in home automation, which is supposed to help people who want to stay at home as long as possible. Research in the field of health and support for aging is considered essential by some of the people surveyed. However, the latter believe that the proposed schemes do not meet their current needs "in part" and are more designed for people with disabilities. At the time of the experiment, the respondents did not feel directly concerned by the technical devices proposed: these people did not feel old. Old age, in their words, is "a feeling, a change of body, wills and life choices".

New technologies are a subject of divergence among some of the people surveyed, as far as their purpose and the conditions of their deployment are concerned, and this in a gendered way. Some of the women surveyed want more thought from designers about the development of technical devices. They express a fear of enslavement. These findings are consistent with those in the scientific literature, in which women surveyed identified the risk of alienation and generally assigned technologies "simply as an object (not a subject)" [JOU 03, p. 71]. They use the technical tools, but "they do not participate in their design and remain outside the understanding of the principles of machine operation" [JOU 03, p. 61]. For the people we questioned, technology is more synonymous with progress, the future, freedom and/or power.

On the side of the research team, differences appear according to disciplinary background. Thus, for the HSS researchers questioned, old age is characterized by "the feeling and acceptance of limits, influenced by the way others see things". The geriatrician argues that "there is no such thing as old age, it is obsolescence that takes precedence". Finally, the ICST researchers show an understanding of old age as a "life stage", when weaknesses in the body lead to new risks and disabilities. Some of them said that the focus group observation changed their view of old age, particularly because of the identity affirmation of the respondents who considered themselves “not old”.

The technologies developed here have aroused the curiosity of researchers from different disciplines and senior citizens. The interest of the actors concerned is therefore essentially based on the “points of contact between the object and the more or less organized interests it arouses” among the people concerned [AKR 88, p. 22]. The users-experts expressed their willingness to continue exchanges with researchers and experimentation with technological devices for home support. They demand respect for their choices, their wishes and their dignity and express their determination to put forward the necessary financial accessibility of technologies for all.

Analysis of the discourse of the people surveyed, on the one hand, and of scientists, on the other hand, shows a complementarity of knowledge, allowing a more global approach to the phenomena studied and the issues to which they relate. In the next part of this chapter, we present the main findings of the reconsideration of a research experience by the different actors involved.

7.3. When experts-users tell researchers where to look

The participation of users-experts and their voice are central to this collaborative action research: they enable the understanding of their needs, expectations and wishes in terms of home support. The controlled environment experiment revealed to some participants potential “commodities”, but the characteristics of the LLSA sometimes hindered them: they likened it to a “hospital” or even an “arsenal” of technologies. Technical tools in general were pointed out as “unsightly”, to the point of being considered stigmatizing for those who “do not identify as ‘old’” [BOU 02].

7.3.1. *Use of human, technical and digital aids by respondents*

The interviews were an opportunity for some respondents to affirm their preferences for seeking human assistance, even if technical assistance was not totally rejected. For these people, the advantage of human assistance is that it allows them to maintain a social relationship and even to consider satisfying an exceptional need in a very individualized way. It also makes it possible to bring "the outside life" into the life of the person being helped. Another argument put forward is that of job retention. The main expressed disadvantage of expressed human aid is that it is ad hoc, unlike technical aids. The unreliability of this type of aid is a cause for concern. However, these aids can be appreciated precisely because they seem to dispense with human relations and interactions and thus with the gaze of the other. For one person, a certain pragmatism resided in the possibilities of applying the functions of a "talking house: practical for the visually impaired". In general, the LLSA is considered very suitable for people with physical or sensory disabilities, but not for people with mental or cognitive disabilities. It would appear that the latter is the most anxiety-provoking for the participants.

None of the persons investigated wears an alarm necklace, although one of them is equipped with one. The explanation given by this 90-year-old woman is the following: "I say to myself, I hope that if I fall down I can crawl to fetch it (the necklace) from my room". This emergency assistance device, in actual use, did not seem to be of particular interest to the respondents. However, concerns in terms of communication tools were very tangible.

The discourse of the people surveyed is rich and reveals differentiated daily uses of information and communication technologies. These people use the computer for administrative procedures, commercial orders, emails, go on social networks (Facebook, Messenger), communicate by visio (Skype), play games (networked or not, such as Scrabble), search on a dictionary or encyclopedia. These users-experts have a smartphone to communicate and use different applications for geolocation, audio description of films, agenda and voice command. The digital tablet is generally used for cooking recipes and looking at family photos. The purchase of these devices, often recent, was recommended by the children or the person's close circle (friends, neighbors, associations for the visually impaired), who also supported the process of taking charge. The difficulties of appropriation expressed generally concern a need to formalize computer knowledge or what the tools concerned allow.

The use of computers, for example, seems to crystallize the respondents' relationship to technology. There are those who like it, those who hate it, those who have been forced to use it or those who have discovered its practicality. We also note those who describe it as a hindrance to family relationships, rather than a facilitator (example of digitally stored photos: you have to wait until someone competent is available to allow access to these photos). Finally, the technical tool is the subject of conversations between friends to exchange information on its operation and applications. The facilities and conveniences offered by technology are sometimes a source of guilt (as in the use of Amazon to order books instead of going to the bookstore). These different reactions are individualized and very closely linked to the trajectory of each person.

Observing and collecting the words of the people surveyed redirected the work of the researchers into another dimension: moving away from the objective of moving from the controlled environment to the ecological environment in favor of a fine and situated definition of precise needs, based on singular experiences. The individualized dimension of these needs, their definition and justification gradually changed the outlines of the study. The comments of users-experts have thus led the researchers to consider the current uses of new information and communication technologies and then to address the projected uses of the technical devices. The researchers started from the LLSA, and the people we interviewed led them into a wider field, where robotics was expanding to include applications of artificial intelligence.

7.3.2. *Projected uses: from voice command to "smart" robots*

The voice interaction during the experiment was appreciated by the participants, who could possibly use it at home. It is seen as a source of fun, a presence, a possibility of support in the accomplishment of daily tasks, remote control of multiple technical functionalities. The humor of talking machines is requested and appreciated (see Siri application). The users-experts who were questioned make the difference between a voice that seems natural to them, compared to a voice they do not like, which they consider to be artificial. The commands addressed to the machine, according to the wishes of the respondents, would be phrased, possibly leading to a dialogue. These people also imagine a personalized robot that they would train to their habits and needs, even to the point of filling a feeling of solitude. One participant – a participant who is *a priori* resistant to information and communication technologies, the use of which has often been imposed on her – spoke of the fact that the machine could be part of her family, in the sense that it would be adopted. Her husband – a pioneer in the use of these technologies – specifies that he would not utter polite words to his eventual robot, because it is not a human. This robot should be equipped with an intelligence that would allow it to understand its environment and to react to it by adapting to it.

For this same participant, more than just home automation objects, it would be the entire house that would need to be automated. So, it would be all the existing features in a house that could benefit from automatic control, rather than individual objects. However, there is a strong expectation that technical objects must not become a constraint for the individual: they must be highly adaptable not only to the individual, but also to his or her environment, to his or her daily life, at the risk of becoming inappropriate. A visually impaired person imagines information and recognition systems (of faces, food labels, room temperature, etc.). Detection and warning systems would also be expected to prevent domestic disasters (water damage, gas, wood stove, etc.) and to ensure the safety of the habitat (closing doors, shutters, gates, etc.).

Finally, the subject of autonomous cars aroused a great deal of interest among respondents. They mentioned these vehicles on several occasions as a possible solution to the loss of mobility or caused by the loss of a driving license. The wishes and hopes expressed reveal a gap between the demand and the supply available on the market for home assistance technologies. The users-experts who were questioned consider that researchers show "good will" in the search for solutions adapted to the needs of people with loss of autonomy. However, they are confronted with known and/or anticipated technical limitations (adaptation of devices to the individual's ecological environment, reliability), as well as budgetary, competitive, legislative, partnership, human and social uncertainties.

7.4. Among researchers: postures linked to disciplinary backgrounds

In these two successive studies, ICST and HSS researchers have developed qualitative and quantitative methodological tools. The overhanging gaze of the trainee in sociology made it possible to study how disciplinary backgrounds underpin different approaches and conceptions of the research subject, for example, with regard to the expression of ethical concerns.

In the course of the risk analysis work initiated by the geriatrician, a reconfiguration of research concerns emerged, leading to a consensus within the team that “technology is not a need, it is a means”. Researchers have therefore insisted on one point: technologies should not create a need, but respond to it. Although risk analysis was not central to the study – at the time of its implementation, it was a matter of familiarizing all the researchers with a working tool – it nevertheless allowed exchanges that were distanced from the pure object of the research and, therefore, allowed team members to take a step back. Thus, the analysis of the methodological risks of a scientific work has become, in the work presented here, a support for the expression of different scientific concerns in the same research field. Observed and analyzed by the sociology trainee, this step back brought out new reflections, questions and positions.

The HSS researchers questioned defended “humanists” concerns, insisting on the notion of respect, benevolence, freedom of speech and mutual understanding with the people surveyed. The ICST researchers interviewed were more concerned with technical and protocol content. The latter insisted on compliance with administrative procedures, security, data retention and anonymization. The issue of intrusiveness was interpreted in a variety of ways: it concerned the technical aspects for HSS researchers (e.g. the presence of cameras); the concern of ICTS researchers was more about their presence in participants’ homes.

The researchers were confronted with very tight temporalities, reciprocal semantic misunderstandings due to heterogeneous disciplinary backgrounds, recurrent unavailability and psychosocial difficulties on a subject as delicate as aging. The distance between the personal and professional spheres has been undermined, making working conditions more difficult, impacting availability for ongoing studies, without this having been anticipated. However, a form of benevolence could be observed between the researchers in these difficult moments: mutual help, asking for personal news, apologies made after some occasional vivid remarks.

A framing of interpersonal tensions and conflicts seems indispensable to maintain the trust gained between researchers and to foster a climate conducive to the production of “a new representation of reality” [DIE 14].

Researchers are thus led to admit the disorder in which science is based, where facts are socially constructed through transformations, translations and displacements – and are not pre-existing to scientific manipulations. Reality is constructed from disorder, which "must be considered the rule and order the exception" [LAT 81, p. 271]. More precisely, "it is thanks to the chaotic dimension of action research that new knowledge emerges, and it is thanks to its structured dimension that it is possible to grasp it" [STO 12, p. 21].

In the field that concerns us, the framing of interpersonal tensions has resulted, among other things, in reciprocal demands: in this study, HSS researchers have strongly forced ICST researchers to adopt a comprehensive stance on needs, with a method of collection and qualitative analysis. The latter asked their colleagues to give an almost masterly and well-argued presentation of the qualitative work, a presentation that aimed to evaluate this singular approach. An "empathy effort" has been created by the members of this multidisciplinary research team, to access the meanings carried by the actors on the desired living environment for the years to come. The researchers recognized the "double punishment" inflicted on the participants through immersion in a controlled environment, on the one hand, and through the imposition of instructions (the execution of a scenario), on the other hand. However, the LLSA offers greater experimental safety than the ecological environment: no risk to volunteers, less uncertainty as to the field of investigation, reliable and high performance technical installation.

The methodological reflexivity of the second study, through the collection of the words of users-experts, aimed to allow each researcher "to be aware of their research, its values and its goals, likely to influence their approach and their interpretations" [MOR 08, p. 35]. It has been fruitful, in that it has allowed research to be redirected towards a thorough study of the actual and projected uses of the proposed technologies in LLSAs.

7.5. Conclusion

This reflexive feedback on two LLSA research projects inspires us to make several reflections. We remind you that it is not exhaustive and specify that the people surveyed were mainly from intermediate socio-professional categories. We have given a large place to the postures of the different actors, as well as to the uses projected by the users-experts: the objective of this research and the methodological tools used brought us to this point… but it is indeed the reconsideration of this work as a whole that has enabled us to identify and deepen the reflection on some of the elements that underlie a whole system. This system included different actors: users-experts, researchers, sociology student trainee; technological objects used in a controlled environment; a mixed qualitative and quantitative approach; the collection and analysis of discourse; real and projected uses, all elements belonging to different registers and implemented in a complex organization.

The postures that emerged in the course of this action research demonstrate, from our point of view, the added value of participatory research, particularly with regard to the orientation and reorientation of scientific work. They also point to some difficulties of cross-comprehension in interdisciplinary research work and allow us to consider the limitations of the LLSA. We have seen that gaps are emerging between institutional expectations and user demands, which open the door to new work perspectives, perhaps through the conduct of longitudinal action research, which would allow a more refined and situated approach to real needs. Interdisciplinarity, which is cumbersome to implement, seems to us to be essential, however: it is a guarantee, through the demands and concerns it interconnects, of permanent questioning and challenges and, therefore, of a form of reconsideration in the work under construction.

In order to decompartmentalize the disciplines and encourage this dynamic, "some do not hesitate to celebrate the organizational chaos, even the surrounding brothel as a breeding ground for innovation" (Roland Moreno quoted by Besnier and Perricault [BES 13, p. 13]) and recognize the serendipity of scientific discoveries. On this point, it seems important to us to recall the centrality of the people surveyed: they are the ones who led the research team to the precise study of projected uses. They were also the ones who insisted on a *sine qua non* condition for the use of technological equipment: the preservation of a decision-making power, which was expressed in particular by the request to benefit from a choice of ordering modalities, instead of looking for the most suitable one. For example, they want to be able to control the opening of the shutters via a tablet while interacting vocally to request that the radio be turned on to a particular station.

In this sense, rethinking research can lead to rethinking the relationship *with* sciences through the relationship *to* science, which is about producing knowledge. The most fruitful and socially useful seems to us to come from work that is accompanied by overhanging, cross-referencing, putting things into perspective and reworking them in a dynamic process of reconsideration.

We would like to thank Véronique Feyfant, sociologist, who participated in the analysis of the interviews used in this chapter

7.6. References

[AKR 88] AKRICH M., CALLON M., LATOUR B., "A quoi tient le succès des innovations? 1: L'art de l'intéressement; 2: Le choix des porte-parole. Gérer et Comprendre", *Annales des Mines*, no. 11, pp. 4–17, 1988.

[AQU 08] AQUINO J., "Le plan national 'bien vieillir'", *Gérontologie et société*, no. 125, pp. 39–52, 2008.

[BER 17] BERTHOU V., PICARD R., "Les Livings Labs, ces leviers d'innovation en santé publique", *Annales des Mines – Réalités industrielles*, no. 2, pp. 68–72, 2017.

[BES 13] BESNIER J.-M., PERRICAULT J., "Introduction générale", *Hermès La Revue*, no. 67, pp. 13–15, 2013.

[BON 08] BONHOMME S., Méthodologie et outils pour la conception d'un habitat intelligent, INPT thesis, Toulouse, 2008.

[BON 13] BONNEUIL C., JOLY P.-B., *Sciences, techniques et société*, La Découverte, Paris, 2013.

[BOU 02] BOUCHAYER F., GORGEON C., ROZENKIER A., *Les techniques de la vie quotidienne. Âges et usages*, DRESS, Paris, 2002.

[CAR 99] CARADEC V., "Vieillissement et usage des technologies. Une perspective identitaire et relationnelle", *Réseaux*, no. 96, pp. 45–95, 1999.

[CLE 16] CLEMENT S., DUBREUIL C., "L'offre technique dans le travail de définition de la vieillesse", *Retraite et société*, no. 75, pp. 17–29, March 2016.

[COE 01] COENEN H., "Recherche-action: rapports entre chercheurs et acteurs", *Revue internationale de psychosociologie*, vol. VII, pp. 19–32, 2001.

[DIE 14] DIEMER A., "Chapitre 4. L'EDD, une initiation à la complexité, la transdisciplinarité et la pédagogie critique", in MARQUAT C., DIEMER A. (eds), *Education au développement durable. Enjeux et controverses*, De Boeck Supérieur, Louvain-la-Neuve, 2014.

[ENN 13] ENNUYER B., "Enjeux de sens et enjeux politiques de la notion de dépendance", *Gérontologie et société*, no. 145, pp. 25–35, 2013.

[FRA 10] FRANCO A., RIALLE V., "Perte d'autonomie et maintien à domicile", *Esprit*, no. 7, pp. 85–92, July 2010.

[GAR 12] GARDIEN È., *Des innovations sociales par et pour les personnes en situation de handicap*, Eres, Toulouse, 2012.

[GOF 64] GOFFMAN E., "The neglected situation", *American Anthropologist*, vol. 66, no. 6, pp. 133–136, 1964.

[JOU 03] JOUËT J., "Technologies de communication et genre: Des relations en construction", *Réseaux*, no. 120, pp. 53–86, 2003.

[LAL 91] LALIVE D'ÉPINAY C., *Vieillir ou la Vie à inventer*, L'Harmattan, Paris, 1991.

[LAT 81] LATOUR B., *La vie de laboratoire*, La Découverte, Paris, 1981.

[LEC 13] LE CROSNIER H., NEUBAUER C., STORUP B., "Sciences participatives ou ingénierie sociale: quand amateurs et chercheurs co-produisent les savoirs", *Hermès*, no. 67, pp. 68–74, 2013.

[LES 15] LES CHERCHEURS IGNORANTS, "Introduction", *Les recherches-actions collaboratives: Une révolution de la connaissance*, Presses de l'EHESP, Rennes, 2015.

[MAR 00] MARCILLAT H., GUILLEMARD A.-M., *Vieillesse et société: le rendez-vous manqué: la dépendance des personnes âgées en question*, Erès, Paris, 2000.

[MAY 17] MAYERE A., "La e-santé et la question des inégalités sociales de santé", in LANG T. (ed.), *Les inégalités sociales de santé: Actes du séminaire de recherche de la DRESS 2015-2016*, Editions Dicom, Lens, pp. 265–275, 2017.

[MEM 08] MEMBRADO M. (ed.), Habiter et vieillir: les âges du "chez soi", Activity report for the fonds National de la science, Université de Toulouse le Mirail, Toulouse, 2008.

[MEM 13] MEMBRADO M., ROUYER A., *Habiter et vieillir. Vers de nouvelles demeures*, Erès, Toulouse, 2013.

[MOR 08] MORILLON L., "Chapitre 2. Recueil et analyse de données en sciences humaines et sociales un panorama", in LELEU-MERVIEL S. (ed.), *Objectiver l'humain? Volume 1. Qualification, quantification*, Hermès Sciences-Lavoisier, Paris, pp. 31–65, 2008.

[NEZ 13] NEZ H., "Savoir d'usage", in CASILLO I. (ed.), *Dictionnaire critique et interdisciplinaire de la participation*, GIS Démocratie et Participation, Paris, available at: http://www.dicopart.fr/fr/dico/savoir-dusage, 2013.

[PAG 14] PAGANELLI C., CLAVIER V., "S'informer *via* les médias sociaux de santé: quelle place pour les experts?", *Le Temps des médias*, no. 23 available at: http://www.histoiredesmedias.com/S-informer-via-des-medias-sociaux.html, 2014.

[POR 13] PORTET F., VACHER M., GOLANSKI C. *et al.*, "Design and evaluation of a smart home voice interface for the elderly: acceptability and objection aspects", *Personal and Ubiquitous Computing*, vol. 17, pp. 127–144, 2013.

[STO 12] STOLOFF S., BEAUDOIN S., "Regards croisés sur la collaboration des acteurs en recherche-action : enjeux et défis", *Recherches qualitatives*, Special edition, no. 13, pp. 20–34, 2012.

[TER 17] TERRAL P., "Participations des patients et des citoyens en santé: l'enjeu de la coordination des expertises scientifiques, techniques et d'usages", in LANG T. (ed.), *Les inégalités sociales de santé: Actes du séminaire de recherche de la DRESS 2015-2016*, Editions Dicom, Lens, pp. 199–218, 2017.

[VIG 17] VIGOUROUX N., CAMPO E., GRIMAUD G. *et al.*, "Approche méthodologique pluridisciplinaire pour l'observation de la prise en main de technologies numériques par des personnes âgées", in PAYRE S. (ed.), *Des services à la personne à la silver économie? Comment accompagner le vieillissement de la population à domicile sur les territoires aujourd'hui et demain*, Chapter 5, Management Prospective Editions, Paris, pp. 103–120, 2017.

8

For a Comprehensive Approach to the Info-communication Practices of Breast Cancer Prevention Stakeholders: A Reflection on Screening

8.1. Introduction

Prevention can be defined as "the set of measures designed to avoid an event that is foreseeable and believed to cause harm to the individual or community"[1]. Anticipating risks is therefore a complex challenge. To do this, a number of players are multiplying "messages" (the information content around prevention) or even "prevention campaigns" (i.e. the system for disseminating messages) in different fields (food, health, road safety, etc.). We note from the outset that there are many actors, which makes it potentially difficult to analyze prevention [MIG 18]. We then postulate that it is first of all a question of identifying and thinking about the actors in their context. Moreover, as prevention is situated, the variables to be apprehended can be varied and makes it more than legitimate to reflect on methodological choices. In this chapter, we reflect, on the one hand, on how to think globally about prevention, and, on the other hand, on the methodological framework for understanding this phenomenon and its info-communication issues. Thus,

---

Chapter written by Dorsaf OMRANE and Pierre MIGNOT.

1 http://www.cnrtl.fr/definition/prévention.

in the case of our research, we are interested in prevention in the context of public health and more particularly in the info-communication practices of the actors (public and private institutions, associations, health practitioners, population concerned) related to organized breast cancer screening.

Our field of research is based on the analysis of one form of prevention: organized screening. We have been working with DOC31 since 2016. This is a *groupement d'intérêt public*, public interest grouping (GIP) in France created in October 2003 whose main financers are the *Caisses Primaires d'Assurance Maladie et l'Etat*, French Primary Health Insurance Funds and the State. DOC31 implements and coordinates organized cancer screening for the population of the Haute-Garonne department in France. Cancer screening is managed at the national level by the INCa (National Cancer Institute in France), the Ministry of Health, the Health Insurance and the InVS (*Institut national de Veille Saniatire)*, French National Institute for Health Surveillance.

In this chapter, we will present the methodological choices of two projects that we conducted using the DOC31 structure. The first project concerns the analysis of two Web-based exchange spaces on organized breast cancer screening (2015–2018). The first is on social networks, notably Facebook with the page of the association "*Le cancer du sein parlons-en*" (Let's talk about[2] breast cancer), which aims to inform and raise awareness about breast cancer prevention [MIG 2018]. The second is the analysis of the consultation process conducted by INCa and mandated by the Ministry of Health in 2016 with the participation of a steering committee of experts, institutional representatives and users. The aim of this consultation is "to initiate a collective reflection on the evolution of organized breast cancer screening" by collecting the opinions and expectations of citizens and practitioners. The online collection of contributions was opened between October 2015 and April 2016 "so that everyone, citizens, professionals, representatives of associations and institutions, can express themselves freely"[3].

2 In 1994, the Estée Lauder France cosmetics group joined forces with *Marie Claire* magazine to find the association "*Le cancer du sein, parlons-en*" *(Let's talk about breast cancer).*

3 https://www.e-cancer.fr/Institut-national-du-cancer/Democratie-sanitaire/Concertation-citoyenne-sur-le-depistage-du-cancer-du-sein#toc-la-concertation-citoyenne-et-scientifique.

The second project (2018–2019) is funded by INCa under a call for intervention research projects in the human and social sciences[4]. Its aim is to analyze the information and communication practices of general practitioners in the Haute-Garonne. It also aims to set up and evaluate an information and communication system for general practitioners. This is a series of short scientific conferences in the form of a literature review addressing the major issues raised by organized cancer screening. Each lecture, not exceeding six minutes in length, shall be prepared by a scientific personality whose work is recognized, from the public or private sector. These lectures will be filmed and retransmitted via a secure website for general practitioners.

In this context, we can see that the two studies mobilize a transversal reflection around the role of the actors (here essentially general practitioners and the population concerned), their representations and their info-communication practices in different contexts related to breast cancer screening. Our work consists of analyzing the methodological choices then adopted. But before that, we begin by briefly presenting the context of organized screening in France.

8.2. State of the art of organized screening, a complex prevention system

While the context of prevention is complex, organized breast cancer screening is no exception. Screening has become a protean object, with a diversity of actors acting within the framework of prevention as well as with controversies and varied stakes.

8.2.1. *Screening: device, issues and controversies*

The programme de Dépistage organisé du Cancer du Sein, DOCS, organized breast cancer screening program in France, presents a plural info-communication system: training for doctors, awareness and information

4 OMRANE D., MIGNOT P., *Dépistage organisé du cancer du sein et médecins généralistes: de la nécessité de reenser le dispositif info-communicationnel*, Activity report INCa Project "Recherche interventionnelle en santé des populations: Agir à tous les temps du cancer", 2019.

workshops, "Pink October" campaigns, mobilization of information and digital communication platforms (Facebook, Twitter, etc.). In France, the DOCS program was launched in 2004. All women over 50 and up to 75 years of age – i.e. 9.5 million women – are thus invited every two years to undergo a mammogram, which is fully covered by health insurance. The issues are important from a public health perspective. More than 22 million mammography screenings have been organized in this way. The five-year net survival rate for breast cancer is 86% for those diagnosed between 1989 and 2004. In 2014, more than one in two women participated in this screening, representing nearly 2,520,000 people. In addition to these figures, approximately 10% to 15% of women perform screening mammograms at the request of the physician or on their own initiative, known as spontaneous, opportunistic or individual[5] screening. Screening, whether individual or organized, is therefore now present in the daily medical lives of women aged 50 to 75. Institutions and information and communication spaces on primary and secondary prevention have multiplied.

For more than a century, breast cancer experts and their institutions have adhered to the principle of early diagnosis and treatment, which organizes the medico-centric standards of screening. However, this unanimity is more and more contested [JUN 03]. In addition, every screening program is subject to debate and, for both the expert and the lay person, there can be many questions in terms of accuracy and safety, for example. How many people are likely to be "false positives", i.e. positive tests in people without the disease, or "false negatives", i.e. negative tests in people with the disease? What kind of effective treatment is available to eradicate the symptoms of the disease being detected? Are these treatments themselves safe? The examination of these questions is nowadays reserved for the judgment of experts in a general way [OMR 18]. In addition, digital social networks offer spaces for exchange to those who offer other forms of expertise, such as the patient sharing his or her life experience. The medical word is therefore no longer the unique and the only accessible on the subject of disease and its prevention.

Although officially implemented throughout France for more than a decade, organized screening was called into question long before it was

5 https://www.e-cancer.fr/Comprendre-prevenir-depister/Se-faire-depister/Depistage-du-cancer-du-sein/Des-informations-sur-le-depistage.

finally established on a national scale. The end of the 1980s saw the first divergent opinions emerge, but it was in 2000 that the controversy really began, and has continued to grow until today. Various researchers and institutions have disproved the usefulness of DOCS through studies establishing its ineffectiveness, while others have refuted previous opinions by reaffirming its usefulness. The media coverage of these discussions between peers reinforces the controversy, ultimately raising the benefit/risk ratio related to this early detection system. A militant movement, outside the medical and health framework, against screening has emerged mainly in the United States [MEN 10] and in France, notably with the publication in 2011 of Rachel Campergue's book entitled "No Mammo: enquête sur le dépistage du cancer du sein" [CAM 11], or the group of doctors "Cancer-rose" who publish on their website the counter discourse on breast cancer screening. Since then, we have seen individual and collective initiatives in France that are moving in the same direction.

The public consultation carried out in France in 2016 brought about these points of discussion, as it is clear that the objectives set at the beginning of the DOCS are hard to be achieved. With ever-increasing year-on-year growth, it was only after four years of running the program at the national level that a stagnation in the participation rate was observed. Intended as a scheme in which nearly 80% of the women concerned (aged between 50 and 75) were to participate, the rates recorded since 2008 fluctuate around 50%. Even if differences can be measured according to territories as well as according to socio-economic groups, the figures are still far from the initial ambitions. Moreover, the questioning of the mortality rate, an indicator used to measure changes in the system, does not argue in favor of the program. Indeed, it is difficult today to assert and prove that a possible decrease in mortality from breast cancer would be directly linked to the presence of DOCS. As mentioned above, the report produced after this consultation also points out the risks associated with screening itself, which can lead to false positives or false negatives, over-diagnosis, over-treatment and certain risks associated with radiotherapy. As a result of this consultation, on April 21, 2017 the public authorities decided on new measures, in particular on information processes, the integration of women over 25 years of age into an information and monitoring system, strengthening the role of general practitioners and gynecologists in the information and awareness raising system, etc. The measures will be implemented by the Ministry of Health.

These measures seem to be aimed at individualized prevention rather than collective prevention, as has been the case up to now. The role of the general practitioner in the DOCS program is thus highlighted as an essential mediator in a prevention system that is increasingly tending towards individualization, even though DOCS remains a national program. This role is all the more important in an uncertain and turbulent socio-medical context [MIG 18].

8.2.2. *Representation of screening: between confidence and mistrust*

Several works in public health and sociology have attempted to identify and possibly understand the obstacles and motivations to breast cancer screening, whether individual screening (DI) or organized screening (DO). These are national [KAL 15] and often local studies. These studies often have as observation criteria or variables social, environmental and/or economic precariousness, culture, biography, the degree of knowledge and information on prevention campaigns, the isolation factor, cancer in relatives or the perception of the practical implementation of screening tests [MAZ 09].

The main motivation for women to get tested would be fear of the disease or the desire to control their health. Those who opt for the DO are confident because of the double reading of the results. Those who opt for DIs consider them to be more reliable than DOs, less anonymous and giving them greater freedom to manage their health [KAL 15]. Often the attending physician or gynecologist plays a decisive role in the choice of screening method.

The observations made by the screening structures, and in particular the one with which we collaborate, highlight a differentiated relationship to screening according to the social origin of the women. This observation is validated by certain studies which also state that some patients' arguments against the DOCS or DI demonstrate their lack of knowledge of them [BER 03, KAL 15]. The women participating in the DI had generally begun mammograms before the age of 50 and continue to do so out of habit as well as a lack of awareness of what the DO could bring to their lives in terms of quality. They also explain that they want to remain independent and manage their own health. They have the feeling that they are being called by the management structure when they want to be actors of their own health.

Finally, those who "know" the DO have a negative image of it. They perceive it as a screening "for the poor", anonymous and less effective. Furthermore, for some studies [MAZ 09], it appears difficult to explain people's behavior in relation to screening using objective variables – as opposed to subjective characteristics of individuals – or even factors identified as facilitating or obstructing access to screening or care.

Thus, factors or parameters that are identifiable as a motivator in one person may not be identifiable as a motivator in another. Certain major themes play a role in the decision to carry out a screening: the relationship to health and the body, sensitivity to prevention issues, the fact of having been affected by cancer, confidence in the doctor, etc. They can shed light on what makes people participate or not. Furthermore, perceptions of breast cancer screening highlight the difficulty of talking to women who refuse any type of screening. The first study we conducted therefore attempts to supplement this literature by analyzing "what is said about breast cancer screening" in online discussions.

In addition to the reasons for participation or non-participation in screening cited in these studies, which are often based on individual factors, the relatively uncertain context of breast cancer prevention shows that cultural, historical and organizational characteristics have an impact on the practices of the population concerned. The discourse of the practitioners and the patient–doctor relationship would help to give the women concerned confidence and provide them with individualized information [AKR 09]. However, while the discourse of practitioners seems reassuring for some patients and encourages them to participate in screening, according to the INCa, the general practitioners who are most confronted with these questions on a daily basis do not seem to be sufficiently involved in the DO program and do not have enough information to position themselves in favor of the DOCS. The second study we conducted therefore explores the perceptions, representations and practices of general practitioners in the context of the DOCS.

8.3. Need to understand the field of screening: methodological framework

As we have just mentioned, the context is complex because it is linked to a tangle of actors (public institutions, health practitioners, private organizations, populations concerned), some of whom are involved in the controversy surrounding screening. In order to record the words of these actors who express themselves and act in a variety of spaces, we use complementary collection and analysis techniques that we question in this chapter. First of all, we have initiated an exploratory quantitative approach that allows us to better understand the actors, the context and the reality of the field we are studying. Two techniques are being implemented: a lexicometric analysis of the content of online exchanges; a questionnaire to general practitioners in the Haute-Garonne, in order to identify their info-communication practices and their perceptions of screening. Then, we adopted a qualitative approach: first with an analysis of the content of the online exchanges of the association "*Le cancer du sein parlons-en*" and of the citizen and scientific consultation; then with interviews conducted on the basis of the findings of the quantitative phase.

8.3.1. *Exploratory approach: quantitative reflection on screening*

Health research on the Internet has multiplied over the past 15 years with the development of digital and mobile technology use by the population and caregivers [THO 13]. A field of study is constituted which is referred to as e-health studies [KIV 13]. Whether quantitative or qualitative, these studies in the human and social sciences make it possible to rethink the relationships between the actors, particularly between patient and doctor [THO 16].

The exploratory quantitative approach seemed necessary to us to first understand the practices related to prevention. Traditionally, quantitative research has focused on accounts and classifications of characteristics and on building models and figures to explain what is observed. In this context, quantitative exploratory research may aim to clarify a problem that is difficult for us to identify as a whole and that is more or less defined. Exploratory research aims for us to circumscribe a space that is too large to be thought of in its entirety [VAN 95]. It is therefore a prerequisite for research which, in order to be deployed, is based on a framework. It thus makes it possible to mark out a reality to be studied in order to collect the most appropriate data. Initially, this research was therefore based on the participation of patients, relatives and various individuals in focus groups. It later became interested in practitioners including doctors.

In the context of the analysis of scientific and citizen dialogue, we have adopted an approach based on data triangulation [OMR 18]. Research on primary prevention issues can combine qualitative and quantitative methods that are mutually enriching. There are many combinations. Qualitative research can precede quantitative research by generating hypotheses to produce and/or test the items in a quantitative questionnaire. Symmetrically, quantitative work can help identify the themes of qualitative research. The two collection techniques can also be used together. It is this last articulation that we have chosen for this study. We have analyzed all open contributions via the Iramuteq lexicometric analysis tool, which is a text and data table analysis software. It is based on the statistical software R and the Python language. Iramuteq offers a set of treatments and tools to assist in the description and analysis of textual corpora and individual/character matrices. We collected text, video and image data. We are also interested in digital traces such as emojis on Facebook and sharing. We also count the number of messages, contributions, likes, shares and subscribers.

In addition, as part of another project with DOC31 financed by the INCa, we have implemented a questionnaire aimed at general practitioners in Haute-Garonne. Its construction was first based on the results of the thesis of Ambre Cazaentre and Pauline Plas [CAZ 16]. They have in fact carried out a qualitative study on the perceptions of general practitioners in the Haute-Garonne on DO, their information needs and their expectations with regard to the management structures of the DOCS. Our questionnaire addresses the themes resulting from the literature review and the analysis of the web content mentioned above: representations of organized screening, organization of the DOCS program, implications of the GP, desired information themes, willingness or unwillingness to participate in the DO system.

This exploratory quantitative research has enabled us to identify the most recurrent themes in the breast cancer screening controversy (over-diagnosis, interval cancers, risks related to mammography, lack of screening assessment, etc.) and also to identify the general practitioner as the main interlocutor in the information and decision-making processes of the population concerned. However, this approach does not make it possible to identify the representations and practices of the various stakeholders. The qualitative approach is therefore essential in a complementary way in our comprehensive approach to information and communication practices related to prevention.

8.3.2. *Ethnographic survey and qualitative content analysis: a comprehensive approach to screening*

The quantitative analysis allowed us to obtain research items to be explored in greater depth and to create an analysis grid for our qualitative approach, which is intended to be comprehensive. The work of Bardin and Kaufman is central to our approach to analyzing web content [BAR 07] and conducting interviews with physicians [KAU 11]. Here, we mean that "the purpose of ethnography is to read a culture as a text in order to understand a body foreign to the researcher" [CLÉ 13, p. 53]. In order to understand the object, we will analyze "a collection of ethnographic reports, characteristic narratives, typical expressions, folkloric facts and magic formulas, must form a corpus that serves as testimony on the indigenous mentality" [CLÉ 13, p. 54]. We seek to understand practices in the info-communicational sense, i.e. representations, uses, behaviors and attitudes in specific contexts. This approach is detailed here in two corpora: the content of digital exchanges on the Facebook page " Le Cancer du sein, parlons-en" and interviews with general practitioners in the Haute-Garonne department in France.

8.3.2.1. *Internet content analysis*

In the first project, we developed a content analysis [BAR 07] on a corpus of contributions from the Facebook page "Le cancer du sein, parlons-en". These allow us to understand and interpret representations that are in the process of being constructed [PAI 11]. This two-year study (2015/2017) gives us the opportunity not to restrict ourselves to a geographical area and to look for the people concerned where they are (the choice of the exchange space). In addition, the possible anonymity allows participants to intervene freely. Finally, this way of doing things opens up possibilities to be in contact with participants in order to complete the study (interview, focus group, etc.). We were interested in two types of content [NEG 06]. First, the manifest content in the sense of what is said explicitly, the themes most often dealt with, the terms that recur frequently, the clear and well-argued or unargued positions taken on the prevention of cancers in general and breast cancer in particular. Next, the latent content, i.e. everything that is not explicitly expressed. Interpretation makes it possible to reveal it from the associative chains. Analyzing latent content then means questioning the absence of a theme or an argument, as well as trying to understand what this absence hides [NEG 06]. With respect to our corpus, we have tried to understand the limited literature and interactions that relate directly and explicitly to the breast cancer screening experience.

For the analysis, we refer to Pierre Paillé and Alex Mucchielli [PAI 12]. They distinguish three modes of content analysis that we mobilize in this work. "Logico-esthetic" analysis studies the structure of discourse in relation to its effects of meaning. This is the case of the stylistic analysis of discourse, which we use in the context of the analysis of the choice of occurrences. For example, analysis of the warrior vocabulary (fight, war, win, defeat, etc.) adopted by some people with breast cancer. Then, the "structural semantic" analysis seeks to define the field of meanings of an object in its context. We would like to analyze the recurrence of the actors, the types of content and the production context, for example, during the "Pink October" campaign[6]. Finally, the "logical-semantic" analysis sticks to the manifest content, considering only the immediate, accessible signified. This analysis focuses on the judgments made by the speaker and the major themes addressed by the actors. The analysis of the controversies was an opportunity to think about actions and reactions in terms of form and substance.

To quote Edgar Morin, the qualitative method approach makes it possible to replace "a thought that separates and reduces with a thought that distinguishes and connects" [MOR 00, p. 21]. It is therefore a "quest for meaning" [PAI 12, p. 13]: "Qualitative data is in fact so multidimensional that only the human mind can hope to extract the most meaning from it" [PAI 12, p. 14]. Pierre Paillé raises here a point that seems important to us: the search for meaning comes from the link we want to have (or create) with the sources. The search for meaning involves finding a less systematic and perhaps more "artisanal" method, i.e. with tools that are not very mechanized. For example, in qualitative analyses, this is the case of persons who do their analyses by hand. In our experience, this has the effect of slowing down the process and thus offers a finer, more attentive sensoriality. This artisanal work also allows a more "carnal" contact with the materials, and consequently "well embodied analyses" [PAI 12, p. 14]. The crossing of sources and especially the search for the specific, characteristic element, which may appear at first glance as a detail, shows the way in which scientists can highlight their corpus. The interpretative approach adopted

6 Annual awareness campaign for the prevention and screening of breast cancer. Initiated in France in 1994 by Marie Claire magazine and the Estée Lauder group.

"implies entering into a renewed relationship with the object of study, which brings together worlds embodied by actors and researchers in the service of an understanding that is still in the process of being formed" [PAI 12, p. 7].

It is with this posture that we have analyzed, over three years, the corpus of the "Le cancer du sein parlons-en" page in a particular context (the "Pink October" campaign). While the quantitative analysis allowed us to identify the key words and most frequent occurrences, the "home-made" content analysis allowed us to identify the links between stakeholders and perceptions of prevention on a longitudinal basis. The major contribution of this analysis lies in the identification of parallel, ubiquitous and highly interactive content on this breast cancer screening awareness space, that of patients. Their words about their life experiences, whether or not they mention screening, are of interest to the population concerned. However, this interest is virtually absent from institutional discourse on prevention and screening. The latter, which is often medico-technical or considered very empowering, is not in line with the practices and perceptions of the population concerned [OMR, 18].

8.3.2.2. *Interviews with doctors*

In the second project, the general practitioner is placed at the center of the screening device. In retaining the interview, we endorse the words of Stéphane Beaud [BEA 96] who assumes the "non-representative" character of this technique. We believe that the exceptional and unique nature of each interview, within the framework of an ethnographic approach, allows us to highlight the singularity and to appreciate the representations of the interviewees.

Thus, restricting the number of interviews is in a way to trust the possibilities of this technique. The aim is to bring out the coherence of social attitudes and behaviors, by inscribing them in a history or trajectory that is both personal and collective. This allows us to detach ourselves from the sometimes frenetic need that prompts the researcher to increase the size of his/her sample. This progressive approach to the field also leads to making pre-selections and choices among possible interviews. Ethnographic research teaches us very quickly that not every social person can be "interviewed" and that there are social conditions for speaking out. In other words: "it must be possible to evaluate, on a case-by-case basis, as an investigation proceeds, the provisional validity of the various investigative techniques available to the sociologist" [BEA 96, p. 237].

The analysis of the interviews revealed the practices and representations of physicians in a context of controversy. Although the majority of the sample interviewed quantitatively by questionnaire is in favor of organized breast cancer screening, the interviews enabled us to identify "discomforts", "annoyed" doctors who are not in control of the controversy, do not inform themselves, trust and apply national instructions or, on the contrary, are critical and multiply their sources of information.

8.4. Conclusion

The presentation of our method would not be complete without an *a posteriori* reflection on the contributions and the limits of the choices made. With regard to the analysis of the info-communication practices of general practitioners within the framework of the organized screening system, the method developed and the initial results are conclusive in the geographical area studied, Haute-Garonne. Thus, the fine analysis of the contents of the interviews allows us to deepen certain findings resulting from the statistical analysis carried out on a larger population. We have, for example, used the questionnaires administered to general practitioners to identify their information resources, the perceived advantages and limitations of organized screening and indicators of reluctance or adherence to it. The analysis of the interviews allowed us to deepen these results and thus to understand, for example, the use or non-use of informational and institutional resources such as those of DOC31 or INCa, as well as individual practices and representations with regard to the organized screening system. Moreover, the combination of an exploratory quantitative and a comprehensive qualitative approach offers us a better understanding of the context, the position of the GP and his or her involvement in the organized breast cancer screening system in Haute-Garonne. But it is legitimate to ask whether such a quantitative/qualitative articulation would be adapted to other areas of prevention? Indeed, we have the ambition to extend our research to other actors (health practitioners) in other territories (the Occitanie region).

Among the limitations of our method, we can first cite the availability and interest of physicians in the study. Depending on their sensitivity for screening, they responded more or less favorably. Thus, our method did not allow access to refractory doctors (those against systematic screening or issuing a critical opinion) and "non-public" doctors. As with any socio-professional practice, so-called "conventional" discourses emerge "naturally" and we have a relative absence of counter-discourse. It must therefore certainly be assumed that they are more present in the public debate than our study reveals. These points of view must therefore be brought together by complementary techniques, such as collecting and analyzing the content of interviews in the press, on forums and Facebook groups fuelling the DOCS controversy, for example. The last limitation of our system, which would also explain the relative absence of counter-speech, concerns the nature of our qualitative sample. Aware of the issue of screening, some of the doctors questioned are also involved in cancerology at different levels: training at the Toulouse Oncopole, participation in research projects, etc.

As far as the content analysis of the corpus of the association "*Le cancer du sein, parlons-en*" is concerned, the method developed and the results are certainly unexpected but prove conclusive. The lexicometric analysis of the page, later supplemented by a more detailed analysis of the interactions during the "Pink October" event, allowed us to consolidate our ethnographic observations online. While lexicometric analysis confirms the virtual absence of the words "prevention" and "screening", it reveals terms that fall within the realm of online social support. Furthermore, content analysis reveals, on the one hand, Corporate Social Responsibility strategies, notably those of the Estée Lauder Group [OMR 16] and, on the other hand, the patient's experiential knowledge (social ties, sharing of experiences, life stories, mediation, etc.). This content, whether implicit or explicit, does not deal directly with breast cancer screening but offers new perspectives on prevention and health promotion in general. Our study could be enriched by interviews with some of the actors involved: community manager of the Facebook page, contributors and readers.

8.5. References

[AKR 09] AKRICH M., MEADEL C., RABEHARISOA V., *Se mobiliser pour la santé: des associations témoignent*, Presses des Mines, Paris, 2009.

[BAR 07] BARDIN L., *L'analyse de contenu*, PUF, Paris, 2007.

[BEA 96] BEAUD S., "L'usage de l'entretien en Sciences Sociales. Plaidoyer pour 'l'entretien ethnographique'", *Politix. Revue des sciences sociales du politique*, vol. 9, no. 35, pp. 226–257, 1996.

[BER 03] BERTOLOTTO F., JOUBERT M., LEROUX M. *et al.*, "Facteurs sociaux de l'absence de participation aux campagnes de dépistage organisé du cancer du sein", *Bulletin Epidémiologique Hebdomadaire*, vol. 4, pp. 24–25, 2003.

[BRA 88] BRABET J., "Faut-il encore parler d'approche qualitative et d'approche quantitative?", *Recherche et Applications en Marketing* (French Edition), vol. 3, no. 1, pp. 75–89, 1988.

[CAM 11] CAMPERGUE R, *No mammo? Enquête sur le dépistage du cancer du sein*, Max Milo Editions, Chevilly Larue, 2011.

[CAZ 16] CAZAENTRE A., PLAS P., Le regard du médecin généraliste sur le dépistage organisé du cancer du sein en Haute-Garonne: étude qualitative par focus groups, Thesis, Université Toulouse 3 Paul Sabatier, 2016.

[CLÉ 13] CLÉRET B., "L'ethnographie comme démarche compréhensive: Immersion dans les dynamiques consommatrices du rap en France", *Recherches qualitatives*, vol. 32, no. 2, pp. 50–77, 2013.

[DEB 00] DE BONVILLE J., *L'analyse de contenu des médias: de la problématique au traitement statistique*, De Boeck Supérieur, Brussels, 2000.

[DUM 16] DUMEZ H., *Méthodologie de la recherche qualitative: Les questions clés de la démarche compréhensive*, Vuibert, Paris, 2016.

[JUN 03] JUNOD B., MASSE R., "Dépistage du cancer du sein et médicalisation de la santé publique", *Santé publique*, vol. 15, no. 2, pp. 125–129, 2003.

[KAL 15] KALECINSKI J., REGNIER-DENOIS V., OUEDRAOGO S. *et al.*, "Dépistage organisé ou individuel du cancer du sein? Attitudes et représentations des femmes", *Santé Publique*, vol. 27, no. 2, pp. 213–220, 2015.

[KAU 11] KAUFMANN J.C., *L'entretien compréhensif*, Armand Colin, Paris, 2011.

[KIV 16] KIVITS J., *Les recherches qualitatives en santé*, Armand Colin, Paris, 2016.

[LAD 08] LADURON I., Approche quantitative et exploratoire des croyances psychologiques, épistémologiques et pédagogiques de futurs enseignants du primaire, University of Liège, Liège, Belgium, 2008.

[MAZ 09] MAZET P., Motifs de participation et de non-participation au dépistage du cancer, Enquête qualitative auprès des habitants de deux territoires de l'agglomération grenobloise, Etude PRéCARRé, Note de travail intermédiaire, available at: https://odenore.msh-alpes.fr/documents/PRECARRE_interm.pdf, 2009.

[MÉN 10] MÉNORET M., "Objets ici, actrices là-bas. Les patientes françaises, passagères clandestines d'un mouvement social du cancer du sein", *Pratiques*, no. 49, pp. 32–36, 2010.

[MIG 18] MIGNOT P., OMRANE D., "Online info-communication practices in the face of a crisis of trust in breast cancer prevention", in PAGANELLI C. (ed.), *Confidence and Legitimacy in Health Information and Communication*, ISTE Ltd, London and Wiley, New York, pp. 107–134, 2018.

[MOR 00] MORIN E., *Les sept savoirs nécessaires à l'éducation du futur*, Le Seuil, Paris, 2000.

[NEG 06] NEGURA L., "L'analyse de contenu dans l'étude des représentations sociales", *SociologieS*, available at: http://journals.openedition.org/sociologies/993, 2006.

[OMR 16] OMRANE D., "Médiation numérique de la Responsabilité Sociale d'Entreprise: prévention contre le cancer du sein", *Revue française des sciences de l'information et de la communication*, no. 9, available at: http://journals.openedition.org/rfsic/2328, 2016.

[OMR 18] OMRANE D., MIGNOT P., "Préventions des cancers du sein: ce que la controverse fait à l'action publique", *Les Enjeux de l'Information et de la Communication*, le supplément 2018A, available at: https://lesenjeux.univ-grenoble-alpes.fr/pageshtml/art2018.html#supplementA, 2018.

[PAI 11] PAILLE P., "Les conditions de l'analyse qualitative", *SociologieS*, vol. 11, available at: http://sociologies.revues.org/3557, 2011.

[PAI 12] PAILLE P., MUCCHIELLI A., *L'analyse qualitative en sciences humaines et sociales*, Armand Colin, Paris, 2012.

[POT 12] POTVIN L., BILODEAU A., GENDRON S., "Trois conceptions de la nature des programmes: implications pour l'évaluation de programmes complexes en santé publique", *The Canadian Journal of Program Evaluation*, vol. 26, no. 3, pp. 91–104, 2012.

[POT 13] POTVIN L., DI RUGGIERO E., SHOVELLER J., "Pour une science des solutions: la recherche interventionnelle en santé des populations", *La santé en action*, vol. 425, pp. 13–15, 2013.

[POY 16] POYET F., GENEVOIS S., "Vers un modèle compréhensif de la généralisation des usages des ENT dans l'enseignement secondaire", *Revue française de pédagogie*, vol. 181, pp. 83–98, 2016.

[THO 13] THOËR C., "Internet: un facteur de transformation de la relation médecin-patient ?", *Communiquer. Revue de communication sociale et publique*, no. 10, pp. 1–24. 2013.

[THO 16] THOËR C., MILLERAND F., "Internet comme terrain d'investigation et mode de collecte des données qualitatives en santé", in KIVITS J. (ed.), *Les recherches qualitatives en santé*, Armand Colin, Paris, pp. 151–164, 2016.

[TRU 06] TRUDEL L., SIMARD C., VONARX N., "La recherche qualitative est-elle nécessairement exploratoire ?", *Recherches qualitatives*, vol. 5, pp. 38–55, 2006.

[VAN 95] VAN DER MAREN J.-M., *Méthodes de recherche pour l'éducation*, Presses de l'Université de Montréal, Montreal, 1995.

9

Health Research on Immunization after 2016: The Need for a Plural Methodological Approach

9.1. Introduction

Following the increase in a climate of mistrust in France with regard to vaccination, which can be observed in a drop in vaccination coverage, the government took up this issue by commissioning a report in 2016. The objective was to provide elements of understanding to the increase in negative positions leading to vaccination refusals, while at the same time contributing to reassuring the general public. Since the submission of this report by Sandrine Hurel at the end of 2016 on the French vaccination policy, several dysfunctions have been identified, including a significant decline in trust among the population as well as among some doctors [HUR 16]. The main actors who suffer from this trust are those in the pharmaceutical sector: “A certain mistrust has developed towards pharmaceutical companies and, even if it is not in the majority, towards vaccination” [HUR 16, online]. However, trust remains central to any process of evolution and change in immunization policy[1].

However, it is important to remember that this loss of trust is widespread in the health system [SAO 09]. This report is also a response to the lack of

Chapter written by Mylène COSTES and Audrey ARNOULT.

1 As Sandrine Hurel points out in her report: “The various studies carried out, publications and hearings have shown that without mutual trust on this subject between institutions, health professionals and users, it is unlikely that the degree of adherence will improve” [HUR 16, p. 91].

visibility of the French vaccination system. Consistency between compulsory and recommended vaccines is not at all understandable, even though this has implications in terms of administration, criminal law and compensation. The aim is therefore to improve the readability and coherence of the policy chosen by the government [HUR 16].

Following this report, a citizens' consultation was set up. It was part of an action plan for the renewal of the vaccination policy issued by the Ministry of Health. The outcome of this consultation (November 2016) recommended increasing the number of compulsory vaccines from 3 to 11[2] on January 01, 2018. In the long term, once trust has been restored, the objective is to have the obligation to vaccinate lifted. The Hurel report refers to "consensual membership". Although no forecast date has been announced, it seems that the target is set for a few years, which implies a legislative vector as well as an assessment of its social acceptability.

Vaccination remains a highly controversial subject, strongly contested by the public, the media and even a minority, but very present, fringe of health professionals. Several studies have outlined the main criticisms made. They concern the dangerousness of the presence of aluminum-type additives, a proven fact, as well as several health scandals (not proven) but which have marked the minds of the population. Several collective fears have emerged about a possible onset of autism or multiple sclerosis. Some high-profile doctors have taken a strong stance against over vaccination, such as Professor Joyeux. Among the opponents or refractory, many are those who denounce the pharmaceutical lobbies or the impossibility of obtaining only the compulsory vaccines, first because of supply difficulties and then by stopping their independent production [AMO 13, BAL 07, CEL 16, GUS 05, LIM 15].

There are several possible explanations for this reluctance. First of all, it should be remembered that many of the diseases against which people are vaccinated today were virtually eradicated until the last few years, which has led to a more distant relationship to risk, although this notion remains at the center of health discourse [ROM 15]. As a result, the counter-effect of medical progress is a decline in immunization coverage and a resurgence of almost forgotten diseases. In this context, the question that arises relates to

2 Comité d'orientation de la concertation citoyenne sur la vaccination, Rapport sur la vaccination, [Online]. Available at: http://concertation-vaccination.fr/category/rapport/, 2016.

both the place and role(s) of information sources in vaccine hesitation, which is defined as "the delay in accepting or refusing [some] vaccines despite the availability of immunization services" [ANG 17, p. 25].

This question arose following a first phase of study [COS 18] and led to a reflexivity concerning the need for a plural methodological approach. This is what we wish to report in this chapter by outlining the methodological course of this research. To do this, we proceed in two stages. We begin by taking stock of the exploratory study by pointing out the methodological questions that it may have generated. Then, we present the methodological construction of the second part of our study by combining the contributions of an analysis by semi-structured interviews and a lexicometric analysis [DUC 14], via the Iramuteq software. Contrary to the first phase of the study, this work aims, above all, to question the need for a plurality of methodologies in health research and to better identify the parameters relating to cases of vaccine hesitation in France concerning children's vaccines.

9.2. An exploratory study that raises methodological questions

9.2.1. *Construction of research questions*

The first part of our study was born out of an exchange with a pediatrician. His questioning was linked to the observation of a drop in vaccination coverage and the difficulty of convincing some parents to have their child(ren) vaccinated. The pediatrician wanted to know the relevant informational elements or devices so that parents would accept the immunization of their child(ren), especially for the optional vaccines, many of which have since become mandatory. We started from the hypothesis of a strong influence of circulating discourses on social networks. The primary objective was to produce applied research to assist physicians and pediatricians with vaccine information.

Beyond our status as researchers, we are also parents. To resolve the issue of distancing, we relied on the notion of "committed neutrality" [HEI 02]. Our initial questions then were: what do we base our trust in our children's health on? How is this trust built and what distribution can be observed among the different sources of information?

9.2.2. *A test methodology with limitations*

The survey was conducted over four days during July and August 2016. A total of 52 people were interviewed by the pediatrician, selected in advance by the pediatrician based on their child's age and their availability to answer the survey following the consultation. Taking place in a pediatric practice, it facilitated access to respondents and promoted acceptance of the interview. The interview guide was administered face-to-face by the researcher. It included a number of open-ended questions, which allowed for an analysis that was essentially qualitative in nature, but with some quantitative variables [COS 18]. The guide was developed in collaboration with the pediatrician, hence the need to find formulations that responded to both medical and information and communication science issues. It comprised four main areas that allowed a progressive entry into the specific and sensitive subject of childhood vaccination: the health information-seeking practices of the respondent (the parent), his or her knowledge and representations of vaccination, his or her access to and approach (if any) to seeking information on vaccination and the forms and interactional content operated on the subject with the various health professionals.

The objective of the study was quickly explained by the pediatrician following the consultation as being research on the subject of childhood vaccination. Given the sensitive nature of the subject, we particularly insisted on the neutrality of the professional's positioning during this presentation. This choice allowed both an optimized acceptance rate and a filter: the pediatrician selected the parents with or without the ability to respond[3]. This bias reveals limits to be taken into account when considering a methodological adjustment. Thus, we perceived that some parents felt constrained and gave very summative answers without any real development. In addition, the place of investigation itself raised questions. It is true that being in a space dedicated to care allows you to focus on the theme of health, but the presence of the child, who is sometimes ill, makes the parent less available. The average length of the interviews was around 20 minutes.

3 For example, parents of children under 2 months of age or showing a certain eagerness were not selected.

9.2.3. *Reflexivity on the concept of "axiological neutrality"*

From the outset of the interview, we saw the need to justify our position as a researcher in information and communication sciences. It seemed important for some respondents to know that we did not intervene at the request of the pediatrician or at the request of pharmaceutical companies. We felt a need for reassurance, for trust building before we could receive the word of these parents. To do this, the method deployed by Nathalie Heinich [HEI 02] in her work on the sociology of controversies was particularly effective. It proposes to distinguish between the researcher, the expert and the thinker. The researcher's position is to be in the understanding and explanation of the social world. The author deploys the concept of "axiological neutrality" to initiate a reflexivity on how to conduct interviews. This is possible and even necessary for research, especially in areas subject to tension, as is the case here, in the medical sector, and more specifically in the field of vaccination. It is defined as "a form of methodical distancing from the values of the actors" [HEI 02, p. 123]. It allows a better understanding of the positions but is in no way incompatible with the researcher's commitment.

The researcher's opinion should be given only after and does not require any evaluative judgment on the subject matter of the research. Heinich calls for an attitude based on moving to opposite worlds:

> "Neutrality, in fact, offers the researcher an ability to move between the different arguments, which enables him to give the actors another viewpoint, another way of giving meaning to their investments and, therefore, of acting on them" [HEI 02, p. 124].

This allows researchers, after the investigation, to position themselves as an expert. Their attitude is then qualified by the propensity to mobilize knowledge to respond to practical demands (in our case, those of the pediatrician). In the subsequent section, we briefly review the main results of this survey phase with the aim of explaining their influence on the method.

9.2.4. *Unexpected results that lead to (re)thinking the method deployed*

The main results obtained during this exploratory phase demonstrated a high level of trust in the health professional's discourse. The unofficial information circulating online did not seem to have a clear impact [COS 18]. We therefore wished to take the results further on this point, which appeared rather atypical in comparison with other work carried out in the health information and communication sciences [ROM 08, ROM 12]. The methodological limitations just mentioned and these initial results led us to modify the research questions. It then became the "vaccine hesitation", which was at the center of the questioning. This can be seen as a manifestation of parents making informed choices [VIV 18].

To do this, the methods of researchers from other disciplinary fields working on health were used. Thus, the model developed by Patrick Peretti-Wattel and Pierre Verger [PER 15] concerning vaccine hesitation could enable us to develop standard profiles that would be used to guide the vaccination discourse, in response to the pediatrician's initial request. A review of the literature allowed them to model the different cases of vaccine hesitation which are linked to two factors: the trust placed in conventional medicine and the degree of commitment to controlling one's health, also known as "healthism", i.e. the "propensity to control one's health behaviors in order to increase life expectancy, using official health information" [ANG 17, p. 39].

In his diagram on vaccine hesitation, the author identifies four positions (see Figure 9.1). First of all, unconditional acceptance (a form of "passive conformism"), which concerns parents who have trust in the healthcare system and immunization. They feel little concern about taking care of their health and therefore unconditionally accept vaccination. "Enlightened acceptance" is "active conformity": patients trust the healthcare system and take charge of their own health. Next comes "rationalized hesitation", which concerns patients who are interested, committed to their healthcare and hesitant about vaccination. Finally, "passive hesitation" refers to parents who do not care about their own health or that of their children. In addition to these four postures, Angelucci and Pierre [ANG 17] add "vaccine opposition" for patients who radically and unhesitatingly oppose vaccination.

The parents we interviewed were mainly in the "informed acceptance" category[4]. However, we did not rule out the possibility that this may have

4 For more details on this point, we refer the reader to the synthesis of the results of the first phase of the study [COS 18].

been a bias because the patient groups were exclusively those of a pediatrician. Indeed, in the cases of active hesitation that we encountered, the parents had already consulted a general practitioner opposed to vaccination or were themselves in favor of homeopathic care. Moreover, those in active acceptance were finally few in number to inform themselves on the subject contrary to the parents in a situation of hesitation. In fact, in the second phase of the study, the profiles of the people in our sample were linked more strongly to the position held in the face of hesitation. Among those interviewed, we observed that those with more education had less knowledge of adverse vaccine reactions. Indeed, they confused real undesirable effects and media polemics that were not scientifically proven. Although this may seem paradoxical, we hypothesized that this finding was the result of a stronger media permeation (from all sources) among the upper social classes. To confirm this point, the method of the second stage needed to compare the type and rate of consultation of sources with the degree of vaccine hesitation shown. According to several authors, the development of online information can contribute to an increase in vaccine hesitation [BET, 10]. In Quebec, researchers have recently established a clear causal link between media controversy and vaccine hesitation [DUB 18].

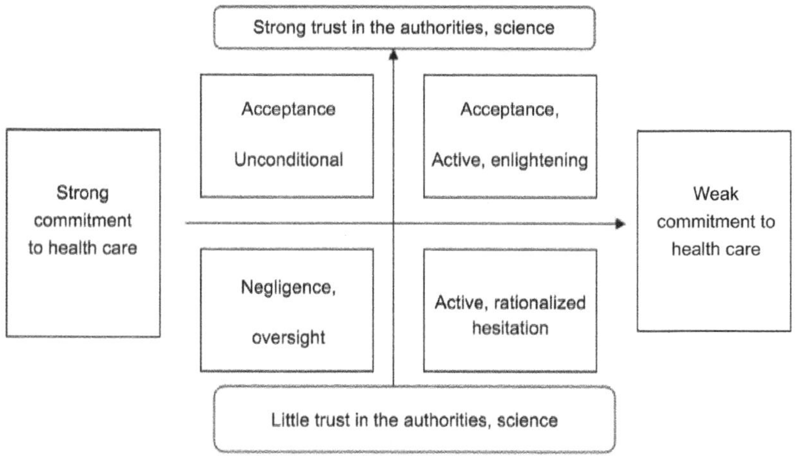

Figure 9.1. *Diagram of vaccine hesitation according to Peretti-Watel and Verger [PER 15]*

For the continuation of our study, it appeared necessary to further the links between socio-demographic profiles, knowledge on the subject and type of vaccine hesitation. In the last part, we present the techniques that seemed most likely to meet the needs of our study.

9.3. The use of lexicometry for the analysis of interviews on vaccine hesitation and opposition

This second part presents the methodological choices we made to continue our study. We explain our questions grounded in the field of information and communication sciences and the techniques of collection and analysis used. In particular, we show how this was achieved.

9.3.1. *Expanded field and themes*

Our main objective was to provide elements of understanding on the issue of vaccine hesitation and opposition. Indeed, the work produced in the medical field often has a practical objective: improving the acceptability of vaccination among parents by giving general practitioners tools to better inform their patients [AMO 13, ENG 17]. In addition, some research was conducted in a different socio-political context, i.e. before the announcement of the change from 3 to 11 mandatory vaccines (summer 2017). The findings of this first phase of the survey prompted us to use a plural method combining semi-directive interviewing and lexicometric analysis. This mixture of approaches (qualitative/quantitative) seemed to us to satisfy our objective. Indeed, while the ontological hypotheses were distinct and induced, *a priori*, differentiated data collection and processing strategies, these approaches were complementary, particularly in order to grasp the complexity of situations. Moreover, particularly for large corpora, quantitative analysis was likely to reveal elements that were invisible to a floating reading and qualitative analysis.

In terms of collection techniques, we used the semi-directive individual interview for its ability to gather rich and precise information as well as to go into greater depth in certain specific areas that were anticipated or that could emerge. To constitute our sample, we wished to identify people in a situation of active, enlightened hesitation or vaccine opposition. To get in touch with them, two techniques were used in a complementary way. Self-administered questionnaires were handed out in both pediatric and general practitioner practices to identify parents in active hesitation or opposition and offered them an in-depth face-to-face interview.

We investigated in both urban and rural settings, as geographical location had been repeatedly shown to be a significant factor in vaccine hesitation [ANG 17, GUI 16]. In addition, we called for testimonials on forums such as Doctissimo. The bias was to only reach people connected and active on these platforms. However, this technique is frequently used in particular on the "Psychology" forum for research on eating disorders, as was, for example, the case with Fleur Bulard [BUL 13]. It has also been, recently, in the context of a thesis on the reluctance to vaccinate [CEL 16].

The maintenance guide covered five axes. The first concerned the representation of immunization both as an individual and as a parent, as the exploratory phase has made it possible to perceive different positions depending on whether it is vaccination in general or vaccination for their child. Then, in a second axis, we addressed the type of vaccination hesitation or opposition. This hesitation could be targeted; it may concern one or more vaccines, and the causes of hesitation may be different for each vaccine. In contrast, the notion of "total vaccine hesitation" applied to all vaccines [ANG 17]. Camille Angelucci and Margaux Pierre point out that:

> "Vaccine hesitation cannot be defined by a single vaccine behavior. It includes different behaviors: non-vaccination, delayed vaccination, and even vaccination according to schedule. A person can vaccinate himself or his child and still have doubts about the effectiveness or usefulness of certain vaccines" [ANG 17, p. 136].

This part of the interview needed to capture the type of total or targeted hesitation and for which vaccine(s), as well as trace the path of vaccine hesitation. Indeed, Patrick Peretti-Watel and Pierre Verger remind us that this path is not necessarily linear: a parent may move from one position to another, but may also have always been opposed to vaccination [PER 15]. This line of study would make it possible to supplement existing knowledge, which mainly reflects the parents' posture at a given time T, without understanding the changes in their position.

A third axis of the interview guide concerned the explanatory factors of these positions. Are these factors medical (side effects, etc.), moral (the question of free will concerning one's health, individual/collective responsibility, etc.), economic or political (the question of the profits of the pharmaceutical industry for example, health scandals, etc.)? To specify this typology of factors, we wanted to cross-reference it with the socio-demographic characteristics of the respondents. Did we see any correlations? Were they identical to those reported in other studies? For Angelucci and Pierre, vaccine hesitation cannot be associated with a lack of knowledge and/or information [ANG 17]. Was it the same for active hesitation as well as for vaccination opposition?

The fourth axis focused on the sources of information that participate (or not) in the construction of this position. The aim was to identify the different sources of information and the trust or mistrust towards these sources. Were there discrepancies between the sources of information mobilized by opposing parents and those used by hesitant parents? Could we identify an evolution of the sources consulted as the path of vaccine hesitation progresses?

Finally, a last axis focused on the role of parents on the forums and the question of the figure of the expert, in connection with studies in information and communication sciences that dealt with health forums [PAG 11, ROM 12, TOU 08, TOU 10]. The questions we asked were as follows: how can discussions on immunization-related forums be characterized? What legitimacy do parents give them? Is it related to the personal experience shared by parents/contributors? Do some parents (or other contributors) play the role of the "lay expert" [THO 10]? We hypothesized that these forums were rather a source of activism for parents who opposed vaccines and/or a place of exchange for those who were in a phase of active hesitation.

9.3.2. *The potential contributions of the Iramuteq software to health research*

The first part of our research was based on a manual analysis of what was said during individual interviews with parents attending a pediatric practice. For this second phase, we wished to use a lexicometric analysis. To use the definition of Lucien Lebart and André Salem, it allowed us to understand "which texts are the most similar in terms of vocabulary and frequency of forms used? What are the forms that characterize each text, by their presence or absence?" [BIA 94, p. 135]. In this, we wish to demonstrate how the use of textual data analysis can be transposable (and relevant) to other research objects in the field of health [LAU 06].

In order to process a larger corpus than with a manual analysis, we used a lexicometric software. As Simon Laflamme reminds us:

> "In some cases, one becomes a way of verifying what has been discovered with the other. In some cases, for example, statistical analysis will have allowed correlations to be established on large samples, while qualitative analysis will allow quasi-experimental observations to be made at the level of individual cases" [LAF 07, p. 142].

It should be noted, however, that lexicometric software has already been used for health research, but mainly on press corpora [JOS 14]. Among the existing software, we retained Iramuteq. It was developed in 2008, within the Laboratoire d'Etudes et de Recherches Appliquées en Sciences Sociales (LERASS – EA 827). A free version of Alceste, it allows you to analyze press speeches as well as interviews, Facebook pages and Twitter accounts. Concretely, different processes allow the software to carry out a formal reorganization of the whole corpus and to conduct statistical analyses on the vocabulary used. For example, it is possible to create word clouds, to work on repeated segments, to identify specificities in contrastive corpora or to determine the themes that structure the discourse.

Among the proposed functionalities, we wanted to use the top-down hierarchical classification for the study of our interviews. This technique allowed us to isolate the main themes of a corpus by a process of fragmentation of discourses into text segments, within which the co-occurring forms were identified [REI 04]. Note that co-occurrence is a "statistically significant association of two items (usually two words) in a given window of text (usually the paragraph)" [MAY 14, p. 18]. It is the recurrent correlation between co-occurring words that gives an overview of the themes present in the speeches. In fact, the co-occurrence of solid words belonging to the same segment can be understood as a possible trace of utterance [REI 07]. The text segments were thus grouped according to the differentiated distribution of their vocabulary, and then gave shape to lexical worlds which were as many thematic universes present in the corpus studied [REI 93]. Each lexical world was materialized by a list of forms, to which was attributed a Chi2 indicating the "coefficient of belonging" of the word to the class. The higher it was, the more important the word was in the construction of the class and for its interpretation.

Technically, the software "makes" a fragmented and nonlinear reading of the corpus. Top-down hierarchical classification is independent of the succession of articles in the corpus, the order of text segments and the order of words. The main advantage of this approach is that it offers a different view of the corpus and brings out elements that the researcher might not have perceived with a simple floating reading, especially for large corpora. In our research, the interest is to be able to associate metadata, at each interview, when coding the corpus. Coding consists, among other things, of choosing the variables that will be associated with the speeches and that will allow the hypotheses to be validated (or not). They must be defined before the corpus is processed by the software and require a good knowledge of the subject and a careful reading of the corpus.

In our research, these variables corresponded to the occupational socio-demographic characteristics of the parents interviewed. They made it possible to characterize discourse and establish correlations between, for example, the criteria of the individuals questioned and the lexical worlds obtained; the types of arguments used to justify the posture of vaccine hesitation (or opposition) or with the sources of information consulted. For example, was there a link between knowledge about adverse vaccine reactions and parental education? These few leads were refined once the interviews were completed, coded and imported into Iramuteq.

9.4. Conclusion

The results considered as significant in the exploratory phase guided the questioning of the research (on the theme of vaccine hesitation), the field (extended to GP practices, online forums and geographically) and the method (enriched with a qualitative/quantitative mix and existing studies on vaccination and/or health in different disciplinary fields). Thus, the approach we advocate in this chapter continuously crosses qualitative and quantitative techniques. For example, while lexicometric software relies on statistical procedures that "appreciate" the distribution of words in texts, it takes into account the "context"[5] and the "co-text"[6]. Moreover, the interpretation of the

5 For example, the speaker, the date, various characteristics, i.e. everything that is metadata.

6 The idea of co-text refers to the notion of co-occurrence. The statistics produced are not a word count. Top-down hierarchical classification is based on the identification of frequently co-occurring forms. A word can be polysemic (the software cannot understand it), but co-occurrence analysis allows us to disambiguate the meaning of this form.

results requires a systematic return to the text and therefore a qualitative "appreciation" of the discourse. This qualitative dimension is also present upstream, during the coding of the corpus, since it is the researcher who chooses the coding variables. The qualitative dimension is therefore present at all stages of the use of this type of software.

Moreover, the method for the second part of our study allowed us to take our first results further, in particular by crossing the socio-professional characteristics of the interviewed parents with the different types of vaccine hesitation. It also made it possible to retrace the path of vaccination hesitation since we presupposed, following Patrick Peretti-Wattel and Pierre Verger, that a parent's position with regard to vaccination can change and is not immutable [PER 15]. What would then be the factors of this evolution? Information sources, type of practitioner, family experience and so on?

From a more general perspective, this research was part of public health work that mobilizes the notion of biopolitics. Proposed by Michel Foucault [FOU 76], this concept was taken up by Didier Fassin and Dominique Memmi [FAS 10a] to designate not only public health policies but also operations of classification, categorization or moralization. The particularity of these mechanisms is that they are not based on intimidation in the name of the law, but rather "substitute an obligation to internalize the norm"; the government of bodies is a government that "makes everyone govern themselves" [FAS 10b, p. 25]. Several health research studies have shown that prevention today is based on the conception of a rational individual who assesses the costs and benefits of his or her own behavior in order to choose (or not) to remedy it [FAS 10b, BER 13]. Did we find elements of this delegated biopolitics in interviews with parents or is the place of the law, via the discourse of health professionals, preponderant?

9.5. References

[AMO 13] AMOUYAL M., VALLART M., BOURREL G. *et al.*, "Que pensent les parents de la vaccination? Une étude qualitative", *Exercer, la revue française de médecine générale*, vol. 24, no. 105, pp. 12–19, 2013.

[ANG 17] ANGELUCCI C., PIERRE M., L'hésitation vaccinale: comportements et attentes. Etude qualitative auprès de médecins généralistes et de patients du Sud-Est de la France, PhD thesis, University of Lyon 1, 2017.

[BAL 07] BALINSKA M.A., LEON C., "Opinions et réticences face à la vaccination", *La Revue de médecine interne*, vol. 28, pp. 28–32, 2007.

[BER 13] BERLIVET L., "Les ressorts de la "biopolitique": "dispositifs de sécurité" et "processus de subjectivation" au prisme de l'histoire de la santé", *Revue d'histoire moderne contemporaine*, no. 60, pp. 97–121, 2013.

[BET 10] BETSCH C., RENKEWITZ F., BETSCH T. *et al.*, "The influence of vaccine-critical website on perceiving vaccination risks", *Journal of Health Psychology*, vol. 3, no. 15, pp. 446–445, 2010.

[BUL 13] BULARD F., Rôle du pharmacien dans la prise en charge multidisciplinaire des troubles du comportement alimentaire, PhD thesis, University of Poitiers, 2013.

[CEL 16] CELLIER C., Réticences autour de la vaccination: analyse des discours des forums de discussion Internet, PhD thesis, University of Lyon 1, 2016.

[COS 18] COSTES M., "Information sources on childhood immunization", in PAGANELLI C. (ed.), *Confidence and Legitimacy in Health Information and Communication*, ISTE Ltd, London and Wiley, New York, pp. 21–38, 2018.

[DUB 18] DUBÉ E., GAGNON D., "Trust, information sources and the impact on decision-making: The example of vaccination", in PAGANELLI C. (ed.), *Confidence and Legitimacy in Health Information and Communication*, ISTE Ltd, London, and Wiley, New York, pp. 61–82, 2018.

[DUC 14] DUCOS A., BONNET V., MARCHAND P. *et al.*, "Classification d'un corpus hétérogène: la page facebook de soutien au "bijoutier de Nice" (septembre 2013)", *JADT, 12° journée internationale d'Analyse statistique des Données Textuelles*, Paris, available at: http://lexicometrica.univ-paris3.fr/jadt/jadt2014/01-ACTES/18-JADT2014.pdf, 2014.

[FAS 10a] FASSIN D., MEMMI D., "Le gouvernement de la vie mode d'emploi", in FASSIN D., MEMMI D. (eds), *Le Gouvernement des corps*, Editions de l'EHESS, Paris, pp. 9–33, 2010.

[FAS 10b] FASSIN D., MEMMI D., "Administrer une matière sensible: conduites raisonnables et pédagogie par corps autour de la naissance et de la mort", in FASSIN D., MEMMI D. (eds), *Le Gouvernement des corps*, Editions de l'EHESS, Paris, pp. 135–154, 2010.

[FOR 07] FORTUNE J., KUMAMAN W., "Préserver les relations avec les parents anti-vaccins, cinq suggestions tirées de la psychologie sociale", *Canadian Family Physician*, vol. 53, no. 12, available at: https://www.ncbi.nlm.nih.gov/pmc/articles/PMC2231532/, 2007.

[FOU 76] FOUCAULT M., *Histoire de la sexualité, Tome 1: la volonté de savoir*, Gallimard, Paris, 1976.

[GUI 16] GUIMIER L., Approche géopolitique de la résistance aux vaccinations en France, Doctoral thesis, University of Paris VIII, 2016.

[GUS 05] GUST D. *et al.*, "Parent attitudes toward immunizations and healthcare providers: The role of information", *American Journal of Preventive Medecine*, no. 29, pp. 105–112, 2005.

[HEI 02] HEINICH N., "Pour une neutralité engagée", *Questions de communication*, no. 2, pp. 117–127, available at: https://journals.openedition.org/questionsdecommunication/7084, 2002.

[HUR 16] HUREL S., Rapport sur la politique vaccinale, Ministère des affaires sociales, de la santé et du droit des femmes, available at: https://solidarites-sante.gouv.fr/IMG/pdf/rapport_sur_la_politique_vaccinale_janvier_2016_.pdf, 2016.

[JOS 14] JOSELIN L. *et al.*, "Dynamiques temporelles de la pandémie de grippe A/H1N1 dans la presse écrite francophone", *JADT, 12e Journées internationales d'Analyse statistique de Données Textuelles*, Paris, pp. 299–310, available at: http://lexicometrica.univ-paris3.fr/jadt/jadt2014/01-ACTES/25-JADT2014.pdf, 2014.

[LAF 07] LAFLAMME S., "Analyses qualitatives et quantitatives: deux visions, une même science", *Nouvelles perspectives en sciences*, vol. 3, no. 1, pp. 141–149, 2007.

[LAU 06] LAUGT O., "Le SRAS dans *Le Monde*: un agent double?", *Les Cahiers du journalisme*, no. 15, pp. 86–101, 2006.

[LEB 94] LEBART L., SALEM A., *Statistique textuelle*, Dunod, Paris, 1994.

[LEB 10] LEBART L., LEJEUNE C., "Montrer, calculer, explorer, analyser. Ce que l'informatique fait (faire) à l'analyse qualitative", *Recherches qualitatives*, no. 9, pp. 15–32, 2010.

[LIM 15] LIMOUSI F. *et al.*, "Les réticences des parents face à la vaccination contre l'hépatite B en France; une enquête en ligne auprès de 5922 parents", *Bulletin épidémiologique hebdomadaire*, nos 26–27, pp. 485–491, available at: http://www.invs.sante.fr/beh/2015/26-27/2015_26-27_2.html, 2015.

[MAY 14] MAYAFFRE D., "Plaidoyer en faveur de l'Analyse de Données co(n)Textuelles. Parcours cooccurrentiels dans le discours présidentiel français (1958-2014)", *JADT, 12e Journées internationales d'Analyse statistique de Données Textuelles,* Paris available at: http://lexicometrica.univ-paris3.fr/jadt/jadt2014/01-ACTES/01-JADT2014.pdf, 2014.

[MOU 12] MOURIER-DUMAS A., Sources d'information et d'influence dans la vaccination, PhD thesis, Jean Monnet University, Saint Etienne, 2012.

[NAB 02] NABARETTE H., "L'internet médical et la consommation d'information par les patients", *Réseaux*, no. 114, pp. 251–285, 2002.

[PAG 11] PAGANELLI C., CLAVIER V., "Le forum de discussion: une ressource informationnelle hybride entre information grand public et information spécialisée", in NASRI LABRIQUE E. (ed.), *Les forums de discussion: agoras du XXIe siècle? Théories, enjeux et pratiques discursives*, L'Harmattan, Paris, pp. 39–55, 2011.

[PAG 14] PAGANELLI C., CLAVIER V., "S'informer *via* les médias sociaux: quelle place pour les experts?", *Le temps des médias*, no. 23, available at: http://www.histoiredesmedias.com/S-informer-via-des-medias-sociaux.html, 2014.

[PER 15] PERETTI-WATEL, P., VERGER P., "L'hésitation vaccinale: une revue critique", *Journal des anti-infectieux*, vol. 17, no. 3, pp. 120–124, 2015.

[RAT 12] RATINAUD P., MARCHAND P., "Recherche improbable d'une homogène diversité: le débat sur l'identité nationale", *Langages*, no. 187, pp. 93–107, 2012.

[RAT 15] RATINAUD P., MARCHAND P., "Des mondes lexicaux aux représentations sociales. Une première approche des thématiques dans les débats à l'Assemblée nationale (1998-2014)", *Mots. Les langages du politique*, no. 108, pp. 57–77, 2015.

[REI 93] REINERT M., "Les "mondes lexicaux" et leur "logique" à travers l'analyse statistique d'un corpus de récits de cauchemars", *Langage et société*, no. 66, pp. 5–39, 1993.

[REI 04] REINERT M., "La méthode d'analyse exploratoire des données textuelles "Alceste" et le problème de l'analyse de contenu", *Les Cahiers de jérico*, no. 4, pp. 79–82, 2004.

[REI 07] REINERT M., "Postures énonciatives et mondes lexicaux stabilisés en analyse statistique de discours", *Langage et société*, nos 121–122, pp. 189–202, 2007.

[REN 07] RENAHY E., PARISOT I., LESIEUR S. *et al.*, WHIST: Enquête web sur les habitudes de recherche d'informations liés à la santé sur Internet, Inserm UMR-S 707, Faculté de Médecine Pierre et Marie Curie, Paris, 2007.

[ROM 08] ROMEYER H., "Tic et santé: entre information médicale et information de santé", *TIC et société*, vol. 2, no. 1, available at: http://ticetsociete.revues.org/365, 2008.

[ROM 12] ROMEYER H., "La santé en ligne: des enjeux au-delà de l'information", *Communication*, vol. 30, no. 1, available at: https://journals.openedition.org/communication/2915, 2012.

[ROM 15] ROMEYER H., "Publicisation et médiatisation des sujets de santé", *Cahiers de l'ILSL*, no. 42, pp. 153–181, 2015.

[ROY 13] ROY N., GARON R., "Etude comparative des logiciels d'aide à l'analyse de données qualitatives: de l'approche automatique à l'approche manuelle", *Recherches qualitatives*, vol. 32, no. 1, pp. 154–180, 2013.

[SAO 09] SAOUT C., "La crise de confiance dans le système de santé", *Les Tribunes de la Santé*, no. 22, pp. 119–132, 2009.

[SAR 12] SARDY R. *et al.*, "Représentations sociales de la vaccination chez les patients et les médecins généralistes: une étude basée sur l'évocation hiérarchisée", *Santé Publique*, vol. 24, no. 6, pp. 547–560, 2012.

[THO 10] THOËR C., AUBE S., "La construction des savoirs relatifs aux médicaments sur Internet: étude exploratoire d'un forum sur les produits amaigrissants utilisés sans supervision médicale", in RENAUD L. (ed.), *Les médias et la santé: de l'émergence à l'appropriation des normes sociales*, Presses de l'Université du Québec, Quebec, pp. 239–266, 2010.

[TOU 08] TOUBOUL A., VERCHER E., "Communication et santé: entre rationalité marchande, logique d'information et communauté d'intérêt", *Tic et Société*, vol. 2, no.1, available at: http://ticetsociete.revues.org/378, 2008.

[TOU 10] TOUBOUL A., VERCHER E., "L'internet santé: stratégie commerciale et développement communautaire", in ROUTIER C., D'ARIPPE A. (eds), *Communication et Santé: enjeux contemporains*, Presses universitaires du Septentrion, Lille, pp. 153–162, 2010.

[VIE 16] VIE LE SAGE F., "Le mouvement antivaccinal: analyse d'un phénomène de société", *Médecine et Enfance*, no. 8, pp. 233–238, 2016.

[VIV 18] VIVON M., "Web 2.0, parenting and informational habitus", in PAGANELLI C. (ed.), *Confidence and Legitimacy in Health Information and Communication*, ISTE Ltd, London, and Wiley, New York, pp. 39–60, 2018.

10

Qualitative Research in Health, in Sign Language: Multimodality and Interculturality of Analytical Work

10.1. Introduction

The conditions of caring for deaf patients are undergoing profound changes, associated with the recognition of sign languages[1] (SL) in the world [KUE 16] and the reforms of health policies and healthcare systems [KAR 15]. Qualitative research in SL in the health field is becoming more diversified. While they share general methodological and ethical reflections [KIV 16], some epistemological aspects deserve to be addressed. After specifying this context and its communicational stakes, we address a few methodological aspects when the languages, media and research samples are different. We discuss the practical conditions for conducting, recording and analyzing interviews in French sign language (FSL), as well as some of the issues involved in publishing interaction analyses in this language. This reflection questions *in fine* the ways researchers participate in the practices they intend to study and on the intermediated and intercultural work in action in the scientific publication of these analyses.

Chapter written by Sophie DALLE-NAZEBI.

1 There are several sign languages in the world that are independent of speech languages. They share a visuo-gestual modality and many linguistic principles that allow us to generalize the methodological issues presented here.

10.2. Topicality of methodological issues in SL research

10.2.1. *Context and issues in SL health research*

Health systems are undergoing a profound transformation redefining the place and voice of patients, who are now seen as "partners" in their care trajectory [KAR 15]. This "democratic transition" of the health system [CHA 16] is associated with an awareness of patients' rights and of a form of "expertise by experience" [EPS 95], which positions patients as legitimate interlocutors in medical research and in the evaluation of the quality of care. Work on this subject in France shows the vulnerability of certain groups for communicational reasons, suggesting the need for linguistic interpretation and cultural mediation in the healthcare system, as well as the necessary adjustment, for these groups, of professional practices and services [JAC 13]. At the same time, the development of a more ecological and interactional conception of disability leads to a reminder at the international level of the right of these people and the need for public services to adapt to them[2].

The relationship to physicians and health is also undergoing a "technological transition" [CHA 16]. The Internet and videos diversify the possibilities of contact and intervention of health professionals (web booking, videoconferencing, telemedicine, etc.). Social media multiply the quantity and diversity of information, as well as the ways in which it can be consulted and discussed. These practices feed into an already long-standing reflection on a public health model based on health promotion communication work. The aim is to involve populations in action on collective determinants (social, economic, educational, environmental, etc.) whose impact on health is now known[3].

This context favors a new attention for deaf people in many countries, including France since the 1990s. Reception and care facilities are set up in the hospital environment by integrating the FSL, through the presence of interpreters and deaf health and mediation professionals [DAG 99].

---

2 The United Nations Convention on the Rights of Persons with Disabilities, ratified by France in 2007, entered into force in the European Union in 2011. http://www.un.org/disabilities/documents/convention/convoptprot-f.pdf.

3 CSDH, *Closing the gap in a generation: health equity through action on the social determinants of health. Final Report of the Commission on Social Determinants of Health*, World Health Organization, Geneva, 2008.

These practices question the specific characteristics of communication on care or health via an interpreter [TIC 15] and via image-based writing[4]. These initiatives require knowledge of the situation and practices of deaf people. They are the subject of surveys on their relationships with the medical world [DAL 08b], on their representations of the body and health, on their levels and networks of information and on their quality of life [SIT 15].

Other initiatives use videoconferencing to make telephone calls (accessible to the deaf) via remote interpretation and in case of emergency calls[5] via direct video communication with agents [DAL 16]. Those who are excluded from the information society would paradoxically be those who could benefit most from it. The policy in favor of access to ICTs for all has become a strong incentive for these audiences to take up ICTs for their own inclusion [DAL 08a]. These innovations, here using SL video, are not just technical; they are transforming the daily lives of deaf people and their relationship to news and social media, as well as the communication and coordination practices of the professionals who interact with them [HEN 13]. They question the communicational, interactional and experiential skills involved in these relationships and new services, raising here the question of expertise, including that of professionals who are themselves deaf [BLA 16].

10.2.2. *The communication dimension at the heart of research activities*

The challenge of the research accompanying these transformations is to have access to the points of view of the interested parties, in all their nuances, as well as to specify the communicational and interactional skills mobilized in these relationships, and therefore to be attentive to the ways of saying and interacting. SLs are visuo-gestual languages, without their own writing system. The recording of speech involves the use of video. These fieldworks reveal in a frontal way the materiality of the researcher's communication practices and investigative techniques. The camera is not one of the usual tools used by sociologists and anthropologists, especially in interviews [TER 85]. The filmed observations, on the other hand, are erased from the research reports, even if they sometimes find cinematic space for

4 Health-BD: http://santebd.org/projet-santebd.

5 National emergency number by video-FSL and real-time text (RTT): http://www.urgence114.fr.

publication [OLI 87]. Workplace studies, conversational analysis and the field of study of mediated communication practices have further explored these issues [HEA 10]. Corpuses in SL are present for the analysis of speech turn-taking management and video communication situations [KEA 10, YOU 12]. These authors are still faced with the question of how to transcribe these data. The signs are transcribed by glosses in the language of the publication text but in the order of production in SL, while a second line of commentary specifies certain modalities of realization. Images from video corpuses are sometimes mobilized. Any transcription or note-taking involves translation. This can supplement the video support in the search process. The majority of SL interview analyses are based on the transcription of their interpretation into the language of the publication. This is not without epistemological and sociological stakes:

> "Qualitative, video-recorded data gathered in/through sign language is mostly translated to the written version of a spoken language. (…) Thus, deaf signers are often studied and represented in ways that ultimately *obscure* the visual, embodied nature of their languages, including their expertise, subjective experiences and participation" [KUS 16, p. 9].

These reflections echo the work on science in progress, encouraging reflective work on intermediate writings and the public presentation of research [SCH 98]. They invite us to question what is negotiated and made visible, within our own scientific frameworks and benchmarks, when speakers of a language without writing are studied, or by people with disabilities. Research in these fields reminds us that scientific rationality "always proceeds in a certain way to enter into communication and to account for this communication" [JEA 04, p.1]. The exploration of these communicational and intercultural dimensions contributes to this reflection called for by Yves Jeanneret "on the researcher's involvement in the communication processes he claims to describe" [JEA 04, p.3].

10.3. The communication challenges of interviews in SL

Here, we need to specify the practical conditions of an interview in SL, and to do so, we must identify the stakes of an analysis work in the source language on video support.

10.3.1. *Challenges of a fine work on what is said in SL*

Offering an interview in SL to deaf people for whom it is the main language, especially via an interpreter, is a remarkable step forward in the world of research. Apart from the silent press, we have no information on what these people lived or thought in France before the 1980s, which saw the birth of a "new social movement" for the promotion of the deaf through participation in FSL [MOT 83]. In its wake, FSL interpreting and teaching professions were structured, long before it was recognized as a language of France by the 2005 law *for equal rights and opportunities, participation and citizenship for people with disabilities.*

In this context, the information given on the interview conditions focuses on the identity of the researcher: whether or not he or she is deaf, whether or not he or she practices a SL [BED 12]. But the majority of social science researchers, including deaf researchers, work from the transcript of the soundtrack of the interview interpretation, either on the day of the interview or on a delayed basis. A thematic analysis from video corpora is possible with various software[6], but this does not avoid the question of citations in the published text.

It is important to underline the difference between interpretation, which involves the oral transmission of a message from one language to another (even from a video), and translation, which is based on fixed media and more faithfully respects the vocabulary, hesitations and repetitions of the source document. The gap between the two does not concern the overall message but the nuances that reflect the feeling and ultimately what is at stake in the testimony. For example, in an interview, a deaf person stated that boarding school in a specialized institute, which was long and with few returns to his home, had cut off his family ties. In this story, he in one instance uses the term "PRISON" to refer to "PENSION", which the interpreter did not immediately spot. This type of nuance gives access to the meaning given by these actors to their experience. This is also shown by the fine analysis of this short excerpt from another FSL interview on suffering at work.

---

6 Let us mention the software "in scope" indexed to the video such as ANVIL, ELAN, NVIVO and those created for the study of SL: SignStream, SL-ANNOTATION. Software such as iMOVIE allows you to label video sequences and various playback modes (slow, fast, "diagonal") of data in SL.

"The problem is that as soon as we get out of meetings, there is a warm exchange of opinions, and I can't take part in that" (Interpretation).

"So, what's the problem with the informal: it's as soon as we get out of meetings, first of all. The hot discussions about what we think, the criticisms, the exchanges, well no, I'm cut off from that. First of all..." (translation).

In addition to the misunderstanding of the expression "*à chaud*" ("without delay"), which here is borrowed from French, the important nuance that the translation introduces concerns the perceived origin of this deaf employee's non-participation in informal exchanges. It is an issue that happens to be at the heart of an uneasiness that is very much shared by deaf people at work: she does not say that this impossibility comes from her ("I can't"), because of a disability, but that she is "cut off from it" by the arbitrary end of the interpretation. This central idea of exclusion and the associated bitterness are perceptible in the details of the realization of the sign "FIRST", which closes this observation. Contrary to the standard sign, where the index finger of the right hand remains resting on the thumb of the left hand (as when counting on one's fingers), the movement of the index finger is here pressed and continued beyond the thumb towards the left shoulder, marking both weariness and ambiguity with another sign whose meaning is "THROW-OUT". However, it opens the beginning of a list of similar situations that ultimately point to the (im)possibilities of participation in a professional collective and the issues of recognition and (loss) of meaning in work.

Working on the source language, from the video medium, allows you to take advantage of visual information on the nature or quality of relationships between groups or individuals. SL is characterized by a syntactic use of space, leading to the arrangement of the entities of the discourse with respect to each other in the so-called signing space, in front of the speaker [CUX 00]. Relational details are provided by the choices of staging. A speaker can show whether or not the working groups, or the types of activities he or she is talking about, are placed on an equal footing; whether or not there was a hierarchical relationship with a particular collaborator; whether or not there were links between these activities and so on. The amount of information actually exceeds the possibilities of simultaneous interpretation. These details are not central to the discourse, but they are decisive in the analysis of experiences, expertise or social relationships.

10.3.2. *Domesticating the camera, keeping your hand on the format of exchanges*

This type of analysis requires access to the original version of the exchange. Introducing a camera into an interview, however, is not without adjustments to normal working practices. It opens up a space for listening as well as for a possible third party to look at the interview and to make public what was said during the interview. If deaf people are used to this tool, its presence raises the question of the use of recording, the framework of the interview and its objectives, especially on health and professional relations issues. Using a camera means introducing questions of consent, image rights and commitment. This works on the relationship of trust between the researcher and their interlocutors. It can be formalized by documents to be signed, in French, raising here again the question of languages and media.

The camera sets up a special formal frame, which is played out as soon as the equipment is installed. The recording marks the beginning and the end of the exchange that is officially part of the interview, words that count. It is common for the interviewee to be concerned about having the camera turned off during a break or sidebar. Associated with this, starting the recording can be stressful because it involves saying things that are worth keeping. The researcher's job is to take control of this tool and the definition of the framework of the exchange, by trivializing this device. It is a question of reappropriating the time and rhythm of interactions by explicitly repositioning the camera as a tool at the service of the researcher, who will be in charge of blanks and other informal times, and will not rush to the camera to cut it off; quite the contrary. He/she will be able to start the recording when the interview objective is recalled. Discussions about confidentiality and image rights can be discussed in front of the camera, which provides a record of them, and decisions about uses can be made at the end of the interview.

The trivialization of this tool does not therefore always involve its invisibility. Researchers have opted to connect the camera to the television set so that everyone can see what is being recorded. Evoking the recording during the interview, concerning what should remain between the interlocutors or concerning the battery, is a reminder that this tool and these traces are at the disposal of the interlocutors and not the other way around. It is through this ostensible trivialization that a space of speech can be protected and a diversity of exchange formats can take place.

Reflections on the paradox of the observer who, through their activity and identity, co-define the situation they observe, do not always lead to a plea for the withdrawal of this observation. Hiding the researcher's intention can make his questions curious and illegitimate; doing without the recording can question what the researcher will ultimately retain from what is said, especially as note-taking is complex here, as listening in SL continuously mobilizes the gaze. This explains why, conversely, the researcher can point out the presence of a camera when it is not detectable, either because the exchange takes place at a distance, in a videoconference, or because the interlocutor is blind or visually impaired in addition to being deaf. In this case, the material is described and presented by touch, in a context where, to capture the nuances of a tactile SL expression (where hands are touched), several cameras may be useful [SCH 09].

10.3.3. *Interacting in SL: a repositioning of bodies and objects*

These SL research practices involve technical and interactional adjustments that highlight the forgotten, because routine, materiality of all communication practices. Beyond the question of equipment, conducting an interview in SL, in relation to a language made of sounds, involves thinking about the relationship to space and repositioning bodies and objects. Communication in SL, when it is not tactile, assumes a distance between the interlocutors allowing each one to see the face, the bust and the whole signing space. It involves maintaining a visual communication link, such as "a thread stretched between two faces" [DEL 08, p.57].

This has concrete implications on the spatial arrangement of the interlocutors and on the management of the researcher's gaze. If the researcher asks for an interpreter, his/her own gaze is free of any constraint and can focus on the interlocutor as well as on their notes. On the other hand, he/she is himself or herself outside the main eye contact of their interlocutor, prompting him or her to verbalize the listening marks transmitted by the interpreter. If, on the other hand, he/she is engaged in listening in SL, the researcher will only be able to look at his/her notes surreptitiously. The management of an interview in SL supposes the memorization of the questions and the formalization of the moments of reading or writing. As leaving the interlocutor's gaze means no longer listening to him or her, this break can only be announced and justified, or be part of a natural break in the exchange. In the case of videoconferencing interviews, where the risk of losing the communication link is increased because it cannot be compensated for by a physical mode of interpellation, the researcher will try to place his/her notes on the same plane as the screen, either by opening a text file on the same interface or by placing his/her sheet on his or her screen. This adjustment of the device makes it easier to move back and forth visually between the notes and the interlocutor, while keeping the interlocutor in his or her field of vision. It recalls the "interdependence of cognitive processes, the use of tools and social organization" [GOO 97, p. 155]; and this gives rise to different configurations depending on the modes of communication and sociolinguistic principles involved. These questions also concern the positioning of the camera, which must keep the two signing interlocutors in its field with a view of the faces, while they are facing each other. The device may also have several cameras whose films will have to be adjusted between them.

This "cognitive ergonomics" shows that the arrangement of bodies and objects in space, and their mobilization over time, takes into account the importance of a visual logic in the management of interactions in SL [LHU 15]. To work in this type of field, the researcher implements interactional strategies and organizational routines that take into account the type of resources and constraints, whether linguistic, semiotic or material. This set of adjustments highlights the fact that professional research practices are based on particular configurations of communication resources. This shift in focus, heuristic in terms of methodology and analytical benchmarks, can pose challenges in publishing work if this experience is not shared.

10.4. Exposing SL speech analysis in publications

10.4.1. *Sharing benchmarks, a professional vision*

Interaction experiments in SL participate in the construction of a "pragmatic analysis grid", in the sense of Bessy and Chateauraynaud [BES 93], i.e. allowing us to identify and give meaning to certain clues leading to the qualification of an object, in this case statements in FSL. It is then possible to report on it from stable and shareable benchmarks, within a community of people. Theses clues and benchmarks equip the researcher's gaze and contribute to a "professional vision" [GOO 94]. But research practices using video and SL are not common. The staging of these analyses in a scientific publication can only partially rely on shared ways of doing and seeing.

This is indeed a common situation in anthropology, since the field is little known. Different strategies are deployed to account for both endogenous practices and logics and the scientific approach to analyzing them. The narration of the research and the use of images and corpus are means to show and understand the work of the researcher in their field [KIL 90]. This contributes to the validation and sharing of the proposed analysis grid. However, the staging of SL research, through translation and images, can update the reference points of a co-verbal gesture and an associated type of reading, making the new reference points proposed difficult to understand. This is shown in the following example from video emergency call drills in FSL, involving 114 officers with deaf college students. They have been analyzed in the context of research on the communication skills of professionals working in SL (especially deaf) in different services.

10.4.2. *Test of an example*

Emergency calls are complex situations of mediatized communication where the agent, although in focused communication with the caller, is required to manage multiple commitments: he/she must complete a form to qualify the request and interact with colleagues to coordinate the emergency response [ZIM 92]. This administrative relationship is marked by relational (between "expert" and "lay person") and interactional asymmetries (these different roles governing the speeches and the themes addressed) [VEL 07]. The video, however, places the officer at the front of the scene and requires that this "public visibility of the body" be taken into account and exploited [GOO 00, p. 1517][7]. The posture and body orientation of the agent, his/her clothing, expressions and gaze, as well as his or her speech and language registers, contribute to setting the framework for interaction, expertise and participation status. They are a reminder of the type of activity that is going on and allow the caller to be seen (or not) as an emergency agent, thus engaging the caller's attention and alignment.

Like other work situations [BOU 01], the management of these calls involves working on and through language. It illustrates the embodied and

7 This is also played out in the publication. We would like to thank the officer, the children and their parents for agreeing to use the images from these PPMS (*Plan Particulier de Mise en Sécurité*) exercises for research.

situated character of any interaction [GOO 00]. But it mobilizes the socially defined rules of interaction in FSL, as well as the linguistic repertoire and semiotic resources specific to this communicational universe, this "visual arena" [TAP 14, p. 132]. The challenge is to understand how officers adjust to their interlocutors, in this case children under stress, in order to be listened to and understood. These situations of mediatized cooperation should make it possible to "demonstrate" the emergency, in a context of asymmetry of information, as well as to "make" emergency gestures, in a context of manipulation of the tablet and collective listening to children in and out of camera[8]. This analysis highlights reformulation strategies that draw on the linguistic repertoire of the FSL. After reporting a student's breathing difficulties, shown on the screen, the agent indicates that the student should be moved to the recovery position (RP) (Figure 10.1). This standard sign is iconic enough to be understood by children: the left hand indicates the ground, and the right hand the body of a person lying on his side.

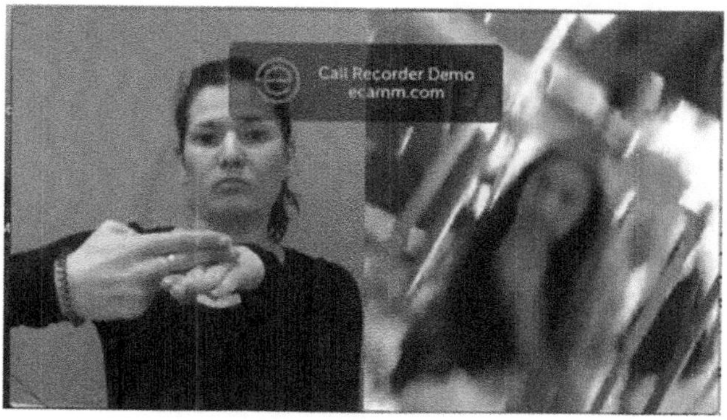

Figure 10.1. *"Putting into RP": first formulation*

Nevertheless, during the exchanges, the agent will formulate this instruction in different ways. The language structures mobilized, known as "personal transfers" [CUX 07], allow us to "say by showing" and to play from different points of view. The first reformulation describes the actions to be undertaken from the point of view of the child helping the other (Figure 10.2); the second endorses the point of view of the victim, grasped

8 We have an internal experimental capture of video exchanges, shown here, and two other views on the platform: one on the workstation, the other on collaboration between agents. The schoolchildren were also filmed in their classrooms, with parents' agreement.

by the hands of her partner (Figure 10.3); the last takes up a position outside the action by using a "proform", a configuration of the hand iconically marking the overall position of the body (Figure 1.4).

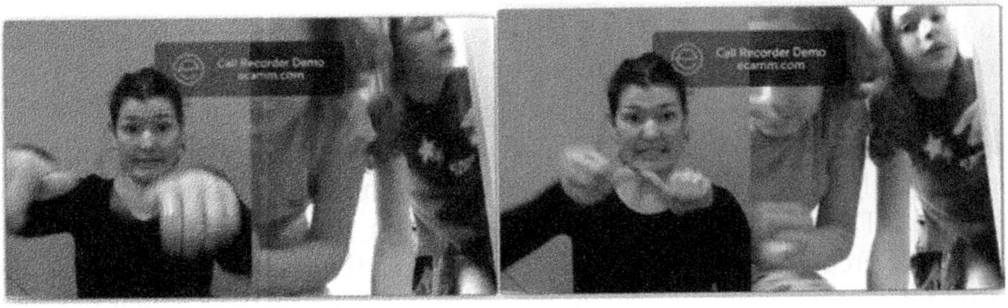

Figure 10.2. *Reformulation 1*

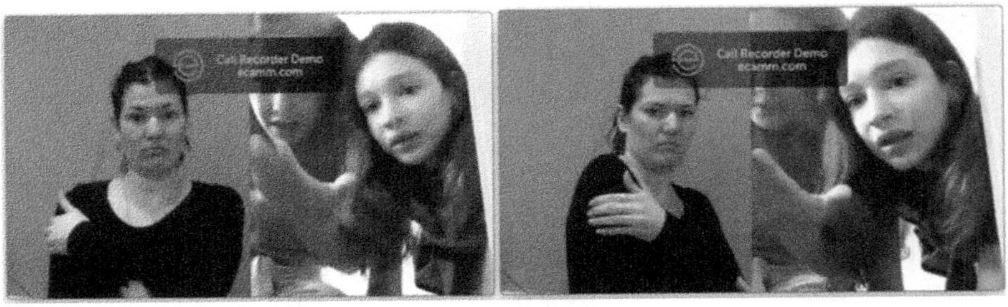

Figure 10.3. *Reformulation 2*

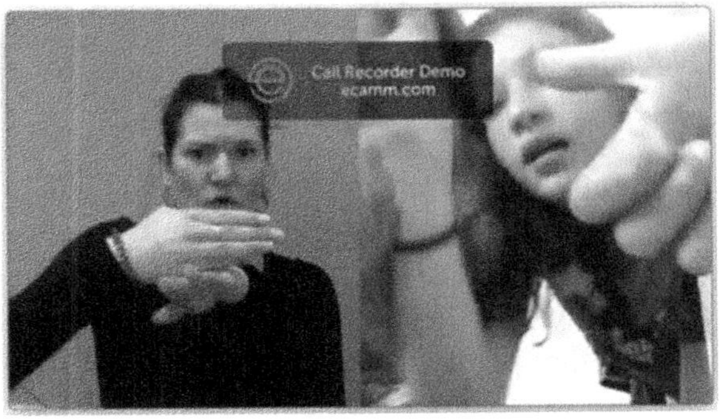

Figure 10.4. *Reformulation 3*

The officer does not take his eyes off his interlocutors during these sequences, which is both a constraint of the emergency relationship (maintaining the visual communication link) and the mark of the prescriptive register in FSL [SAL 03]. Non-prescriptive personal transfers, common in narratives, are marked by the absence of eye contact, with the speaker embodying the character he or she is talking about, expression included. A brief occurrence of this type of transfer can be seen here (Figure 10.5: IM1-3), when the officer describes the child's clumsiness to help point out what needs to be done. A translation of the sequence is shown above. The square brackets indicate correspondence with the images, which illustrate only part of the statement.

> "You, [you think it's okay to put your legs together] IM1. [But you're surprised to see his top leg is tipping over] IM2 [and his body with] IM3. You have to take the leg and [move it over the other one there] IM4".

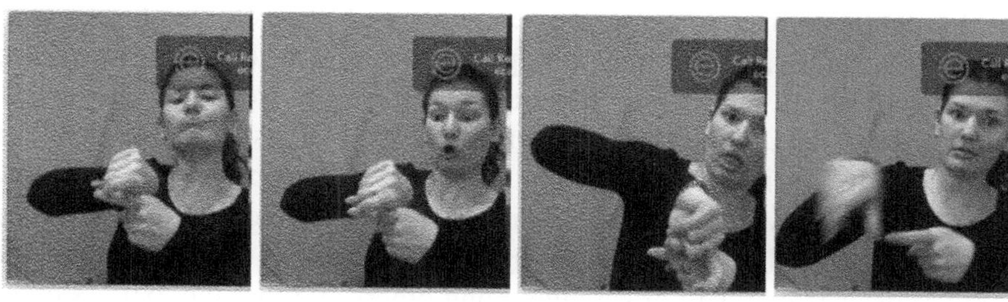

Figure 10.5. *Wrong and right way to put in RP*

The analysis of these excerpts (about 10 seconds in total) highlights the linguistic and interactional work in action, as well as shows the linguistic forms involved. A reader unfamiliar with SL is marked by the importance of facial expressions, which seem emotionally charged, and by expressive forms of mime or co-verbal gestures. Interactions in oral languages are not devoid of gripping gestures as in the reformulations presented. The complexity of these structures, and their linguistic character, is not directly perceptible or understood. This iconicity is, however, "compositional" and linguistic, as this linguist points out:

> "Each parameter involved in the realization of the whole, i.e. direction of the gaze, facial mimicry, as well as the manual components that are the configuration, orientation, location and movement of the hand(s), carries meaning (they are indeed morphemes) both independently (because they are detachable and/or switchable) and depending (the value of each one is a function of its supporting context) on the others" [CUX 07, p. 122–123].

The finesse of this officer's linguistic and interactional work may therefore remain misunderstood. The publication of interaction analysis in SL implies thinking about its "audience" and the possible readings in this space.

10.4.3. *The communicational anchoring of reading*

The publication of images from corpuses in FSL, combined with their written translation, reactivates interpretative cues where emotional and emphatic gesture comes to illustrate, support or regulate the word. The words in FSL are in fact materialized by a translation, written and distinct from the image, which in turn carries descriptive emotions and gestures: as in co-verbal gestures. This makes it invisible that the translated discourse is entirely carried by the gestures present in the image, that the iconic register is one way of saying among others and that the expression of the face and the engagement of the body are linguistic processes. They can be activated, accentuated or relatively neutralized, depending on the register and language repertoire. It all depends on the interactional context, as shown by the cases of asides, in FSL, between colleagues and an officer always in video link with a caller. The signs made by the agent are produced with one hand, out of the camera's field of view, in a low position; the engagement of the bust is neutralized and the facial expression controlled, so that the caller does not see the discussion between professionals[9]. This remains an uncomfortable situation and under severe constraints. However, these variations in body expression and engagement show that they are part of codified and differentiated linguistic and interactional practices.

9 The break in communication between the agent and the caller is visible by the loss of eye contact; it is also explained by a request for hand hold.

The reactivation of reading cues, which are rooted in the practices of languages made of sounds (and co-verbal gestures), makes invisible the professional skills of these agents, who were at the heart of the analysis. The public presentation of field research in SL requires an intercultural effort to explain the linguistic, sociolinguistic and interactional references specific to the SL used. This work encourages us to focus on the semiotic resources that can be mobilized, as well as the relationship to space, bodies and objects specific to the different communicative universes, which are the universes of interaction in vocal languages and SL. This intercultural work on ways of saying, doing, interacting and coordinating in SL is all the more crucial since SL makes partial use of common interaction practices and semiotic resources with vocal languages, but according to different principles and in different registers. It is not only the scientific categorizations of linguistic phenomena that are being challenged but also the more common categorizations of people speaking in languages made of sound, which most researchers and readers are.

10.5. Conclusion

We have highlighted the issues and pragmatic questions raised by methodological approaches that pay attention to the details of the speeches and interactions in the language of the respondents, in this case SL. We have insisted on the decentration brought about by the modality of this language, by a visual logic of interaction; by iconic, spatial and corporal linguistic resources and by the use of video as a medium of analysis. The heuristic scope of the methodological reflections undertaken is to encourage a pragmatic approach to communication issues, taking into account the materiality of communication practices, whether it is a mediated communication or not. This notion of materiality is not limited to the simple consideration of the modalities of communication. It also concerns the arrangement of bodies and objects in space, the management of gaze, touch and expression, as well as a certain geography of exchanges and interactional spaces. It invites us to question the materiality of our analysis tools and devices, in a context where they equip and support a professional vision.

All research engages a representation of scientific work by mobilizing, and staging, certain clues and analytical practices. These benchmarks structure scientific publications, which readers must then understand and share [CHS 98]. The case study of research in SL fields mentioned here invites us to extend this reflection on the materiality of communication practices to the graphic and codified space of writing and reading that is scientific publications. As Souchier, Jeanneret and Le Marec [SOU 03] have reminded us, these imply a "knowing how to read", which is also a "knowing how to take", a practice, which can be learned and which is part of a larger cultural set of ways of doing and seeing. However, it is other reading benchmarks that the researcher reporting on SL must tackle, by working on or questioning the contextual configuration of the resources that are publications. "Thus it becomes impossible (...) to develop knowledge without thinking about its publicity" [JEA 04, p.3] and without thinking in this process of the importance of certain communicational and cultural reference points.

10.6. References

[BED 12] BEDOIN D., "Une ethnographe entendante dans le "monde des sourds": conditions d'enquête auprès d'enfants sourds signeurs", *Les Sciences de l'Education*, vol. 45, no. 4, pp. 15–33, 2012.

[BES 93] BESSY C., CHATEAURAYNAUD F., "Les ressorts de l'expertise. Épreuves d'authenticité et engagement des corps", *Raisons pratiques*, no. 4, pp. 141–164, 1993.

[BLA 16] BLANCHARD J., "Intermédiateurs sourds: un travail sur la communication et les relations sociales", *Actes des Assises nationales de l'inclusion professionnelle et de la diversité, sourds et entendants au travail*, available at: http://www.fnsf.org/wp-content/uploads/2016/07/Assises_Vendredi_ Innovations -Ordinaires-1.pdf, 2016.

[BOU 01] BOUTET J., "La part langagière du travail: bilan et évolution", *Langage et Société*, vol. 98, no. 4, pp. 17–42, 2001.

[CHA 16] CHAMBAUD L., "Le système de santé français à l'épreuve des transitions", *Socio*, no. 6, pp. 157–170, 2016.

[CUX 00] CUXAC C., *Les voies de l'iconicité*, Ophrys, Paris-Gap, 2000.

[CUX 07] CUXAC C., "Une manière de reformuler en langue des signes française", *La linguistique*, vol. 43, no. 1, pp. 117–128, 2007.

[DAG 99] DAGRON J., *Sourds et soignants, deux mondes, une médecine*, In Press, Paris, 1999.

[DAL 08a] DALLE-NAZEBI S., "Technologies Visuelles et e-inclusion. Initiatives de sourds", *Innovation: The European Journal of Social Science Research*, vol. 21, no. 4, pp. 353–369, 2008.

[DAL 08b] DALLE-NAZEBI S., LACHANCE N., "Sourds et médecine: impact des représentations sur les conditions d'accès aux soins. Regards croisés France-Québec", *Interrogations*, no. 6, pp. 78–94, 2008.

[DAL 16] DALLE-NAZEBI S., MADEC A., "Rendre les appels d'urgence accessibles aux sourds. Enjeux d'une articulation entre sociologie et ergonomie", *InnovatiO, revue pluridisciplinaire en innovation*, no. 4, available at: https://innovatio.univ-grenoble-alpes.fr/indexc637.html?id=371, 2016.

[DEL 98] DELAPORTE Y., "Le regard sourd. Comme un fil tendu entre deux visages", *Terrain*, no. 30, pp. 49–66, 1998.

[EPS 95] EPSTEIN S., "The construction of lay expertise: AIDS activism and the forging of credibility in the reform of clinical trials", *Science, Technology and Human Values*, vol. 20, no. 4, pp. 408–437, 1995.

[GOO 94] GOODWIN C., "Professional vision", *American Anthropologist*, vol. 96, no. 3, pp. 606–633, 1994.

[GOO 97] GOODWIN C., GOODWIN C.H., "La coopération au travail dans un aéroport", *Réseaux*, vol. 15, no. 85, pp. 129–162, 1997.

[GOO 00] GOODWIN C., "Action and embodiment within situated human interaction", *Journal of Pragmatics*, no. 32, pp. 1489–1522, 2000.

[HEA 10] HEATH C., HINDMARSH J., LUFF P., *Video in Qualitative Research: Analysing Social Interaction in Everyday Life*, Sage, Los Angeles, 2010.

[HEN 13] HENAULT-TESSIER M., DALLE-NAZEBI S., "TIC et relation administrative. Repenser l'activité, co-construire l'accessibilité", in PATESSON R. (ed.), *Transformation des organisations; Évolution des problématiques et mutations fonctionnelles*, Publication du Centre de Sociologie des Organisations, Collection EUTIC n°7, Brussels, pp. 261–270, 2013.

[JAC 13] JACOB P., Un droit citoyen pour la personne handicapée; Un parcours de soins et de santé sans rupture d'accompagnement, Report, mission auprès de M.A. Carlotti, ministre chargée des personnes handicapées et de la lutte contre l'exclusion et M. Touraine, ministre des affaires sociales et de la santé, available at: http://solidarites-sante.gouv.fr/IMG/pdf/rapport-pjacob-0306-macarlotti.pdf, 2013.

[JEA 04] JEANNERET Y., "Analyse communicationnelle et épistémologie des sciences sociales : Introduction", *Études de communication*, no. 27, pp. 1–7, 2004.

[KAR 15] KARAZIVAN P., DUMEZ V., FLORA L. *et al.*, "The patient-as-partner approach in health care: A conceptual framework for a necessary transition", *Academic Medicine*, vol. 90, no. 4, pp. 437–441, 2015.

Postface

Although they share similarities, in terms of the info-communicational questioning of the relationship between health and the digital world, the chapters in this book report on work carried out in different directions. They do so with different objectives, analytical frameworks and approaches. They demonstrate, if need be, the complexity of the phenomena at work and the value of mobilizing a diversity of fields, approaches, methods and disciplines to undertake some of the contemporary changes. By contextualizing and then methodically describing practices, their issues and sometimes the strategies of the actors involved, the authors do not approach digital technology in its technical dimension alone, avoiding the social or human issue. They postulate that it is first and foremost the product of human rationality and intelligent thought, the expression of a bond between individuals. Their approach therefore focuses, above all, on the systematic description of human uses that integrate the social framework of interactions between humans and machines [PRO 02]. By listing representations, interactions and power relations, they seek to account for the lived experience and to understand what individuals do with digital technology.

The reflexive stance on research approaches, which is the particularity of the book, enables, among other things, the emergence of original questions in the relationship between knowledge and practices. For example, it sheds light on some of the tensions between professional and research practices, especially when the latter is involved, applied and/or responds to a request. Moreover, the intellectual introspection that the authors have shown reveals,

Postface written by Laurent MORILLON.

in a more or less explicit way, their beliefs regarding gnoseological, methodological and knowledge validity issues [PIA 67]. These are therefore epistemological perspectives that transcend the chapters, affirming by the same token what makes knowledge and its value. In terms of health and digital technology, these choices can contribute to ideological struggles [BLA 02] regarding the consideration of humanity and technology, their respective places in society, etc. with regard to a dominant liberal and productivist model that considers technology as one of its sources of development.

The reflections on ethics, first of all, remind us of the extent to which research activity must be guided by moral and democratic concerns [JEA 04], especially in the field of health. It is a question of developing science with concern for oneself, others and the community as a whole [GOM 96], in other words by recognizing in all others an alter ego [GOS 92]. And while it is rare to be able to accuse a humanities and social sciences researcher of willful malice, applied and action research can potentially result in encroachments on the freedom of others. It therefore seems essential to further develop the reflections on researcher distance from the subjects, the subject and whoever ordered the research [BÉZ 96], on the responsibility of the researcher and therefore on the scope of his/her work, on the import of scientific concepts into practice, on the potentially manipulative processes of discourse mobilizing a technical-scientific popularization and mythifying science [CAS 01].

Finally, the reflections on methods demonstrate the richness of the available techniques and their articulations for developing knowledge about health and digital world. The choices made reflect their belonging to the category of "movement science" researchers [LEL 08]. Even more so when they favor qualitative approaches, they postulate the primacy of human and social facts, understood as phenomena of meaning, i.e. as bearers of meanings conveyed by actors involved in an inter-human situation [MUC 02]. What is knowable is therefore ultimately the human experience of reality [VON 01]. The context, which is not considered constant, is studied, described and analyzed. Research then becomes a situated and contextualized activity that can only be established in the context of an interaction between a knowing subject and a phenomenon through a sensitive and then cognitive experience. But this interdependence between the phenomenon and the scientist, this annihilation of the "objective" distance to the object, is likely to generate reservations about the validity of the knowledge thus produced. From the perspective of a study funded by national agencies, or carried out with doctors and/or researchers in the so-called "exact" sciences, it can encourage the adoption of quantitative techniques and propose original articulations.

In the health field, regarding the complex and evolving phenomena resulting from a diversity of influences, injunctions and constitutive interactions, it would be valuable to carry out further research to expatiate on those gathered in this book and in this collection coordinated by Viviane Clavier and Céline Paganelli. More than ever before, social sciences and humanities researchers are relevant to shed light on the long-term relationships of power, the interdependence of issues, permanent adjustments and underlying perspectives. Their involvement through applied research or actions is likely to contribute in an even more significant way to the dissemination of a distanced, or even critical, thinking, in order to fight against preconceived ideas, readiness to think, "fake news" and other alienating discourses from the promoters of technology, control or management. And their words will be all the more credible if they make visible the research "in progress" and open the "black box" of the scientific process.

References

[BÉZ 96] BÉZILLE H., VICENTE M., "La recherche en train de se faire: entre rigueur et compromis", in FELDMAN J., FILLOUX J.-C., LECUYER B.-P. *et al.* (eds), *Ethique, épistémologie et sciences de l'homme*, L'Harmattan, Paris, pp. 173–194, 1996.

[BLA 02] BLANCHARD P., RIBEMONT T. (eds), *Méthodes et outils des sciences sociales*, L'Harmattan, Paris, 2002.

[CAS 01] CASELLAS MENIERE M.-F., "Le travail des doubles", in MACKIEWICZ M.-P. (ed.), *Praticien et chercheur. Parcours dans le champ social*, L'Harmattan, Paris, pp. 55–69, 2001.

[GOM 96] GOMEZ L.-E., "Culpabilité et implication", in FELDMAN J., FILLOUX J.-C., LECUYER B.-P. *et al.* (eds), *Ethique, épistémologie et sciences de l'homme*, L'Harmattan, Paris, pp. 48–58, 1996.

[GOS 92] GOSSELIN G., *Une éthique des sciences sociales. La limite et l'urgence*, L'Harmattan, Paris, 1992.

[JEA 04] JEANNERET Y., OLLIVIER B., "Faire des Sic: praxis, méthodes, pratiques", *Hermès*, no. 38, available at: http://hdl.handle.net/2042/9437, 2004.

[LEL 08] LELEU-MERVIEL S. (ed.), *Objectiver l'humain? Volume 1. Qualification, quantification*, Hermès-Lavoisier, Paris, 2008.

[MUC 02] MUCCHIELLI A. (ed.), *Dictionnaire des méthodes qualitatives en sciences humaines et sociales*, Armand Colin, Paris, 2002.

[PIA 67] PIAGET J., *Logique et connaissance scientifique*, Gallimard, Paris, 1967.

[PRO 02] PROULX S., "Trajectoires d'usages des technologies de communication: les formes d'appropriation d'une culture numérique comme enjeu d'une société du savoir", *Annales des télécommunications*, no. 57, pp. 180–189, 2002.

[VON 01] VON GLASERSFELD E., "The radical constructivist view of science", *Foundations of Science*, special issue on Impact of Radical Constructivism on Science, vol. 6, nos 1–3, pp. 31–43, 2001.

List of Authors

Audrey ARNOULT
LERASS (EA 827)
Paul Sabatier University – Toulouse 3
France

Emilie BLANC
LERASS (EA 827)
Paul Sabatier University – Toulouse 3
France

Elizabeth BOUGEOIS
LERASS (EA 827)
Jean Jaurès University – Toulouse 2
France

Michèle CARIA
LERASS (EA 827)
Paul Sabatier University – Toulouse 3
France

Benoît CORDELIER
ComSanté
UQAM, Université du Québec à Montréal
Canada

Mylène COSTES
LERASS (EA 827)
Jean Jaurès University – Toulouse 2
France

Elodie CRESPEL
CIMEOS (EA 4177)
University of Burgundy – Franche-Comté
Dijon
France

Sophie DALLE-NAZEBI
LERASS (EA 827)
Fondation Maison des Sciences de l'Homme
Paris
France

Erik DE SOIR
Department of Scientific and Technological Research Royal Higher Institute for Defence
Brussels
Belgium

Adrien DEFOSSEZ
LISST (UMR 5193)
University of Toulouse
ISIS, Institut National Universitaire Champollion
Castres
France

Stéphane DJAHANCHAHI
CIMEOS (EA 4177)
University of Burgundy – Franche-Comté
Dijon
France

Olivier GALIBERT
CIMEOS (EA 4177)
University of Burgundy – Franche-Comté
Dijon
France

Hélène GERMAIN
LERASS (EA 827)
Paul Sabatier University – Toulouse 3
France

Claudia Veronica MARQUEZ GONZALEZ
Psychology and Education (CA-98)
Faculty of Psychology
University of Colima
Mexico

Philippe MARRAST
CERTOP (UMR 5044)
Paul Sabatier University – Toulouse 3
Tarbes
France

Pierre MIGNOT
LERASS (EA 827)
Paul Sabatier University – Toulouse 3
France

Laurent MORILLON
LC2S (UMR 8053)
University of the French West Indies
Schoelcher
Martinique
France

Dorsaf OMRANE
LERASS (EA 827)
Paul Sabatier University – Toulouse 3
France

Aurélie POURREZ
CIMEOS (EA 4177)
University of Burgundy - Franche-Comté
Dijon
France

Hélène ROMEYER
CIMEOS (EA 4177)
University of Burgundy – Franche- Comté
Besançon
France

Silvia Rosa SIGALEZ RUIZ
Attached LERASS (EA 827)
Psychology and Education (CA-98)
Faculty of Psychology
University of Colima
Mexico

Index

S, T, U

Other titles from

iSTE

in

Health Engineering and Society

2020

BARBET Jacques, FOUCQUIER Adrien, THOMAS Yves
Therapeutic Progress in Oncology: Towards a Revolution in Cancer Therapy?
(Health and Patients Set – Volume 2)

PAILLIART Isabelle
New Territories in Health
(Health Information Set – Volume 3)

2019

CLAVIER Viviane, DE OLIVEIRA Jean-Philippe
Food and Health: Actor Strategies in Information and Communication
(Health Information Set – Volume 2)

PIZON Frank
Health Education and Prevention
(Health and Patients Set – Volume 1)

2018

HUARD Pierre
The Management of Chronic Diseases: Organizational Innovation and Efficiency

PAGANELLI Céline
Confidence and Legitimacy in Health Information and Communication (Health Information Set – Volume 1)

2017

PICARD Robert
Co-design in Living Labs for Healthcare and Independent Living: Concepts, Methods and Tools

2015

BÉRANGER Jérôme
Medical Information Systems Ethics

Printed and bound by CPI Group (UK) Ltd, Croydon, CR0 4YY

15/09/2026

14962351-0001